The Catholic Guide to Expectant Motherhood

THE VERY REVEREND MONSIGNOR
GEORGE A. KELLY

Director of the Family Life Bureau of the Archdiocese
of New York
Author of The Catholic Marriage Manual *and*
The Catholic Family Handbook

ROBERT J. WALSH, M.D.

Assistant Attending Obstetrician and Gynecologist
St. Vincent's Hospital, New York
Fellow of the American College of Obstetrics
and Gynecology

A. J. VIGNEC, M.D.

Medical Director, New York Foundling Hospital

ROBERT P. ODENWALD, M.D.

Former Professor at Catholic University, Washington;
Author of Your Child's World

Edited by John and Ellen Springer

THE
CATHOLIC
GUIDE
TO
EXPECTANT
MOTHERHOOD

RANDOM HOUSE, NEW YORK

618.2
S 769

NIHIL OBSTAT
John A. Goodwine, J.C.D.

Censor Librorum

IMPRIMATUR

✠ Francis Cardinal Spellman
ARCHBISHOP OF NEW YORK

The nihil obstat *and* imprimatur *are official declarations
that a book or pamphlet is free of doctrinal or moral
error. No implication is contained therein that those
who have granted the* nihil obstat *and* imprimatur *agree
with the contents, opinions or statements expressed.*

. . . .

August 12, 1961

Contents

8 PRAYERS FOR EXPECTANT MOTHERS 195

A prayer for help to become a good mother / A prayer for the privilege of motherhood / Blessing of an Expectant Mother / A Novena to Our Lady of a Happy Delivery.

9 THE EXPECTANT MOTHER'S RECORD 201

A section where you can list phone numbers of your doctor, hospital, pharmacy, and others to be called in an emergency / Pages to record your progress each month and the instructions your doctor gives you on each visit / Space where you may list questions to ask your doctor / By keeping these records, you will be able to compare your progress in later pregnancies with that of your first one.

The Catholic Guide to Expectant Motherhood

1

Motherhood: Your Call to Greatness

The Very Reverend Monsignor GEORGE A. KELLY

*Director of the Family Life Bureau of
the Archdiocese of New York;
Author of* The Catholic Marriage Manual *and*
The Catholic Family Handbook

YOU HAVE BEEN TOUCHED BY GOD

When the great sculptor Michelangelo completed his statue of
Moses in Florence in 1504, he stood back to admire its beauty.
Filled with awe by the precision of every line and the lifelike
quality of every curve, overwhelmed by the beauty of his own
creation, he let his hammer fly at the statue and commanded:
"Speak!" But Moses, magnificent though he looked, did not
reply. He had no power of his own. More than four hundred
years later, at the Roman Basilica of St. Peter in Chains, recognized as one of the greatest of man's achievements, gazed upon
by throngs of admiring tourists, he still sits mute.

Very soon you, an expectant mother, will produce a work of
art incomparably greater than the greatest of Michelangelo's
works: a living child. Compared with your son or daughter, all
the world's sculpture pales into insignificance.

Do you realize what has happened to you? How you have
been blessed by God? What opportunities await you?

Not even the sentimentalist or the cynic can diminish the magnificence of motherhood. The mother who cradles in her arms a newborn child is moved, not with the pride or violence of Michelangelo, but with the humility that comes with the realization that she—more than man—is an intimate partner with God in the wonderful work of creating a human being. What is more divine than the power of creating life? Think for a moment what this means. The hand of God has reached out of Heaven to touch your body in a special way, to give your cells joined with your husband's that individually created living soul whereby your child can breathe, grow, feel, think, love, rule, have mercy, and go back to God from whence he came.

What a privilege is motherhood! To become by divine election an intimate collaborator with God in creating a new being whose life story will never end! God did not need you to bring human beings into the world. He had an endless number of possibilities to choose from. But He *chose* your pregnancy and your childbirth to create the child He wanted born and He elected you as the specific vehicle whereby this "miracle" would be accomplished. This collaboration is your unique benediction. "Blessed art thou among women."

Think a little further. The child you are now carrying depends on you as he depends on no one else. Without you he might die or live as an emotional cripple. This child is like a reed easily shaken by the wind, like a flower from which even the softest breeze plucks some petals. Who gives strength to this delicate reed? Who protects this flower? You. If, as psychologists tell us, the early years of life are the most important to manhood or womanhood or Christian development, then to you does God look—and your child unknowingly does, too— for your solicitude, concern, love, direction and formation.

Your opportunity for supernatural love. Your pregnancy, apart from its contribution to God's Kingdom and to a little infant, will not leave you unchanged, either. Bearing a son or daughter will make you capable of a greater love than you ever believed you could have. Henceforth, your willingness to devote yourself entirely to the service of another human being will constantly amaze you. You will achieve higher levels of mercy, tenderness and compassion than you have ever known before. You will pass through the difficulties of pregnancy and understand what is meant by a "labor of love." Upon the birth of a child, young women frequently experience a change that might almost be called miraculous. Before the hand of God touched them, they may have been inclined to selfishness, always catering to their own self-interest, more concerned with their own comforts and convenience than with anything else. With the experience of motherhood, however, they are transformed. Now, no task is too menial, no sacrifice is too great.

Your husband, too, profits from your motherhood. His tender care of you becomes more pronounced. His pride in the fruitfulness of his love for you is enhanced. To him, henceforth, you become the source, the nourishment and special bulwark of family joy and peace. You enlarge the scope of his affection, bind the father in the love of his children. Mutual love of husband and wife becomes incarnate in a son or daughter. It is purified. It grows. It becomes more spiritual. Pope Pius XII once remarked to newlyweds: "Give us a mother who feels deep within her heart her spiritual as well as natural maternity and we will see her the heroine of the family, the strong woman, whom you can praise in the song of King Samuel in the Book of Proverbs:

"Strength and beauty are her clothing, and she shall laugh in the latter day. She hath opened her mouth to wisdom, and the law of clemency is on her tongue. She hath looked well to the paths of her house, and hath not eaten her bread idle. Her children rose up and called her blessed; her husband, and he praised her.

"Protected by her own industry and good repute, she greets the morrow with a smile. Right wisdom governs her speech, but it is kindly instruction she gives. She keeps watch over all that goes on in her house, not content to go through life eating and sleeping. That is why her children are the first to call her blessed, her husband is loud in her praise: Unrivalled are thou among all the women that have enriched their homes. Vain are the winning ways, beauty is a snare; it is the woman who fears the Lord that will achieve renown. Work such as hers claims its reward; let her life be spoken of with praise at the city gates." (Prov. 31, 25–31.) *

Perhaps the exalted role assigned to you in life terrifies you. But remember, you do not work alone. God, as your original Partner, continues to offer you the graces to be a successful mother. Since in His Kingdom on earth, you represent the Church, you are an instrument of His grace to all around you and you will be supported by Christ Who is the source of all grace. Your activity in the "little Church" of your home will be done on a supernatural level. You work for love—not because the work is pleasant, but because it must be done for Christ's sake. You are like the nun who tenderly washes the disfigured face of the leper. She is motivated not by mere natural sympathy but rather by her love of Christ. She thinks not of the awful face but rather of the fact that her act is pleasing to her Savior.

Never underestimate your ability to be a successful mother.
When God confides a child to the care of a Christian mother, He seems to say to her what Pharaoh's daughter said to the mother of Moses: "Take this child and rear him for me." Probably the most important work of a mother is not child-bearing but child-training. And no one will have greater influence on him than you. He will know no greater.

* *Translation by Monsignor Ronald Knox.*

Your husband ordinarily will dominate a significant part of the child's education—particularly in areas of law and order, family tradition, intellectual attainments, vocational matters, worldly and practical affairs. But in your child's emotional and spiritual development—a development which is more important for his happiness on this earth and in the next—he will reflect what you are. Therefore you will have the power to produce more good in your children than anyone else in this world.

There are two reasons for this. First, the early years of life are decisive for the formation of character. Someone has said: "Everything experienced for the first time in the child remains forever." And his most traumatic early experiences—love or harshness, confidence or fear, piety or impiety—will be with his mother. Secondly, the young child, boy or girl, is very much like a woman, immensely personal, impressionable, imaginative, emotional. And it is the womanly nature of the mother that makes her the teacher par excellence. Her very femininity is the source of her greatest power. Little children drink in with eagerness the lessons they learn from the one who is the source of their life and also of their nourishment.

A mother, then, must prepare herself for this sacred, serious, and solitary mission—sacred because God has delegated her, serious because no art or profession is more difficult and strenuous than that of molding properly the tender soul of a child so easily disfigured, solitary because no one can fully substitute for her.

The Christian mother ought to embrace this opportunity with joy. The grace of matrimony gives her inner strength to perform this task. In her parenthood not only is the child born, but through her child she is also born as a mother. The whole supernatural fabric of the home is built around her. As Pope Pius XII has said: "Precisely in her material mission of child-bearing lies the secret to the mother's salvation and sanctification. A cradle consecrates the Mother."

The Christian mother clings to the vision of her sacred partnership with God. She trusts in Him and in the future. She is not swayed by momentary discouragements. She is confident that her child will achieve his spiritual destiny of eternal life. She knows that by taking human nature from a woman and by exalting His mother, Christ dignified, glorified and sanctified motherhood. She remembers, too, that beneath the Cross, it was the men who turned away. The women stood. Even in this moment of seeming defeat, they knew that all would end well and that the crucified Savior would rise again.

In fulfilling the major role of your life—that of helping your child to lead a happy life during his days on earth, to save his soul for all eternity, to find and play his rightful role in Christ's Mystical Body—you need never worry for a lack of experts to advise you. You can learn much from them about the techniques of child care—about feeding and bathing your youngster and performing all the other tasks which are necessary to keep him well nourished, warm and comfortable. You can also learn much about satisfying his spiritual and emotional needs.

But never forget one thing: You, yourself, are often the best judge of your baby's needs. Regardless of your own educational attainments, God has appointed you to oversee the child's spiritual and emotional development. You—just by being a capable Christian mother—will show him how to view life, how he is God's son as well as yours, what habits of mind and virtue he must possess to please God and render his earthly days valuable. In the true Christian home, more good is done him than in any other way. By your daily actions you show him that you love and serve God, obey the Commandments and practice the virtues. This is the best training ground for meeting the problems of life.

Such parents need not worry unduly about the "right" way to bring up their children. Once the will of God becomes the governing force in your house, you and your children will all

know what is expected of you. They will know that certain acts
are acceptable because they conform to God's laws—and certain things are forbidden because they violate His laws. In
learning to obey and respect His authority, they will learn
to respect your authority as His representative. And in learning
at an early age that wrongdoing brings punishment, they learn
a principle which will guide their conduct all their years and
will even determine whether their lives are judged to be worthy
of reward in the eyes of God.

Why the mother is the heart of the family. The Church has
many names for the mother. Pope Pius XII called her the "sun"
of the family. He expected the Christian mother to diffuse light
and warmth in her home. Her self-sacrificing generosity
spreads love. Her cheer dispels the clouds that overtake many
family days. Her gentility softens the tumults, her simplicity
moderates passions, her power and strength give energy to all
who live with her in God's domestic sanctuary.

Pope Pius XI called her the "heart" of the family. He meant
to imply that just as the heart is vital to good health in the
physical body, so is the mother the center of her husband's and
children's spiritual life.

The heart provides lifeblood and oxygen for the other organs
of the body. Without that blood and without that oxygen,
neither hands, nor feet, nor lungs, nor even the brain, could
function. The mother, too, performs her duties for the good of
others. She often sees the results of her efforts only in the
actions of her husband and her children. She is the hub around
which the family universe revolves. Her vitality invigorates all
others and binds up all wounds.

The heart is an instrument of purification. Through its
operation, impurities in the blood are cleansed. Only by return-
ing to it does the blood retain its life-maintaining function.
So with the mother. She is the seat of love. The husband looks

to her to remove the turmoils and petty difficulties of family life. The children run to her for consolation, support, medicine. Without her purifying example of devotion, family health would languish.

The heart is probably the strongest organ of the body. Under severe attack it shows remarkable capacities for recovery. Physicians often are amazed when they observe a heart that seems to be determined, against all odds, to carry out the function for which God intended it. Does this not describe the good mother? She does her duty even under impossible conditions. She fills the gap left by a father frequently preoccupied by the struggle of making a living. I know one mother, periodically abandoned by a drunken and half-crazed husband, who brought four aggressive sons through the turbulence of their early years until today, in the twilight of life, she contemplates with satisfaction a priest, a doctor, a college professor and a policeman, all the work of her sturdy hands and heart.

The good mother may be driven by disappointments to the point of despair, but she does not give up. Perhaps all others will find fault with her child, even condemn him, but she will stand by his side. No matter what misfortunes befall the family, she will continue as the source of hope for every member.

The measure of a man is the size of his heart. His courage, leadership, magnanimity, daring, kindness are what make him admired and loved. Most truly human values are associated with the heart. History books and encyclopedias, governments and corporations, may pay tribute to a man for his intellectual accomplishments, but people esteem others mostly for the understanding, consideration and affection they manifest.

And these values, when they do come to a man, come chiefly from his mother.

Pregnancy is an ideal time for meditation. Your present state of pregnancy offers an ideal opportunity to draw closer to God.

You may have more time to think about your purpose in life now than you will have for many years to come. You may now consider in quiet solitude why God gave you this life and what He expects of you.

Now, too, is a time to strengthen your religious practices. Frequent reception of the Sacraments, frequent recitation of the Rosary, the conscientious saying of morning and night prayers—all of these will strengthen your faith and strengthen your will to perform your work of motherhood in a satisfactory way.

Meaning of the Blessing of an Expectant Mother. You can obtain special graces in the Blessing of an Expectant Mother. It is a ritual of the Church that is rich in tradition and in blessings. Ask your parish priest to bestow it upon you. In this ceremony, he will offer prayers for your protection and for the welfare of the child God gave you the power to conceive. The full text of the Blessing of an Expectant Mother is contained in the appendix.

At the time of the baby's Baptism, you might also arrange with the priest to give you the traditional Blessing of a Mother after Childbirth. This too is a simple ceremony. Mother and child are met by the priest at the church entrance and led to the altar, where prayers of thanksgiving are said for the gift you have received.

Make the Blessed Mother your own model. Devotion to the Blessed Virgin is especially appropriate at this time. It is she who can best serve as your intermediary in Heaven, and it is she—by virtue of her own motherhood—who is the perfect model of sanctity and sacrifice.

When Mary first heard that she was to be the mother of the Messiah, she too was filled with forebodings and anxiety, and with doubts that she would be able to fulfill the role which

God asked her to play. But then she committed herself to the task with her entire being. She gave herself with a total generosity. And from that time forward, she devoted herself with joy to the tasks that lay ahead.

Like all mothers, she was to know moments of happiness and of sadness, and finally she was to see her Divine Son crucified. But in all the moments of her life, she had a sense of the Divine purpose—an ideal that enabled her to stand above the natural problems of motherhood. She was able to bear her great sorrow because she knew that it furthered the Divine Will.

You too will experience joys in your child. They will not be the sublime joy of the Virgin Mother who knew that her Infant was the son of God. You will know sorrows. They will not be her supreme sorrow in witnessing His death upon the Cross. Nevertheless, you will have moments of travail which may require all of your human strengths—and more—to cope with. You will need God's help to meet your problems. But you too will stand above the natural pains and problems of motherhood if you too give of yourself with a total commitment and a total generosity.

There is good reason to regard the Divine Mother as your model—as the model of patience, gentleness, and understanding, the model of motherhood who willingly made any sacrifice because she was furthering God's work and performing God's will. To the Angel at the Annunciation, she made the response which you might make now and throughout the years to come when you will hold your child's welfare in your hands. She put aside all her doubts and reservations and turned herself over to God. She said: "Be it done according to Your Word."

When she made her decision to give herself completely and absolutely to the work God asked her to do, she took the step which truly was necessary before all generations could call her Blessed. This was her moment of Magnificence, for when she dedicated herself to accept this role, she took a unique position among all the beings who have ever walked on earth.

Now is the time when you too must make decisions. You must decide what kind of guidance you will give your child, what ideals you will hold up to him, what goals in life you will encourage him to seek. If you are true to your beliefs, you will stand before him as an example of sanctity and goodness. There will be no doubt of the objectives he will seek, no doubt of the eternal destiny that will be his. This is your moment for decision. Like that moment when Mary totally committed herself to her task, this is your time for greatness.

WHAT YOU SHOULD KNOW ABOUT YOUR CHILD'S BAPTISM

During your pregnancy, you will probably make two decisions involving the spiritual welfare of your child—the choice of his sponsors in Baptism, in which he becomes a Christian, and your choice of the saint after whom you will name him.

In the normal course of events, most Catholic parents prepare to have their infants baptized by the priest within a month or so after mother and child return home. Of course, if there is any danger to the infant—miscarriage while you are pregnant or serious illness after birth—you should have him baptized immediately.

Anyone can baptize, and the ritual is simple. It consists of pouring water upon the head of the person to be baptized while pronouncing the words, "I baptize thee in the name of the Father, and of the Son and of the Holy Ghost." Most of us memorized this procedure in childhood.

Even if an infant received emergency Baptism, a formal baptismal ceremony must be performed later in your parish church. This ceremony has an important spiritual meaning. The child's godparents (or their representatives) should be

present and he will be given the Christian name he will carry
all his life.

Requirements for godparents. Probably well before the expected birth date, you and your husband will begin to consider candidates to serve as godparents, and you will also begin
to think about a suitable name.

What is the purpose of godparents? As you know, Baptism
is the Sacrament which implants an indelible mark on the soul
and makes us Christians and members of the Mystical Body of
Christ. Our Lord taught that Baptism is necessary for salvation:
"Unless a man be born again of water and the Holy Ghost, he
cannot enter into the Kingdom of God." Unless a person receives Baptism, he is unable to gain all the graces which flow
from that Sacrament. Nor can he receive the other Sacraments
instituted by Christ.

Since this Sacrament is necessary for your child to enjoy the
gift of Faith, it is the foremost one he can receive. He cannot
receive it unless he renounces the devil and his works, and
expresses his determination to follow the teachings of Our
Lord and to lead a true Christian life. Since your infant is unable to speak for himself, the godparents have the responsibility
of expressing that willingness and determination for him.

In speaking for the child, the godparents also promise in effect to make the child's spiritual welfare their concern all their
life. In a practical sense, they probably will not have to do much
in this regard, for your child's spiritual welfare will be primarily
your concern. But if you or your husband should prove unable
to care for your child spiritually, his godparents have the duty
of doing so. In rare cases, they may even be morally required to
make great sacrifices to enable your child to reach adulthood in
a Chirstian environment.

Because godparents undertake a great responsibility, you
should choose them with care. Knowing what is expected of

godparents, you can appreciate why the Church insists that they fulfill several requirements:

1. They must be at least fourteen years old. This is indeed the minimum age at which they could be expected to concern themselves effectively with your child's spiritual welfare if it became necessary to do so.

2. They must be baptized Catholics who now practice the Faith. Obviously, persons who do not receive Penance and the Holy Eucharist as required by Church law, are not practicing Catholics. They can hardly safeguard your child's religion when they jeopardize their own.

3. They must be free to become your child's spiritual guardians if necessary. For this reason, priests or brothers or sisters in religious communities cannot be sponsors unless their superior gives them special permission.

Although the Church does not set a maximum age for godparents, logic suggests that sponsors be young enough so that they might be expected to live until your child is able to care for himself. For this reason, grandparents—unless comparatively young—are not the ideal choice for the office.

It is common practice to name both a godfather and godmother. However, Church law states that you need have only one sponsor. This may be either a man or a woman.

Nor must godparents be present at the Baptism. They may be "godparents by proxy" and have someone represent them. Thus you might choose sponsors who would be unable to attend the ceremonies. They need only write to you indicating their willingness to accept the office, and stating that they meet the necessary conditions for eligibility.

How to choose a suitable name. Church law regarding the choice of a name for your child is equally reasonable. It states: "Pastors should take a special care that a Christian name be given all whom they baptize. If they cannot do this, they shall *add to the name given by the parents, the name of some saint and enter both in the baptismal records." It follows that you should select a name which has some spiritual significance.

A suitable name should not be difficult to find. There are literally hundreds of names for boys and girls for you to choose from. A representative list is given in chapter 7.

The Christian name you select need merely be derived from a saint's name. It may be a variation, a translation into English, or a diminutive. Since many names have a dozen suitable variations, the choice is great.

For example, the name Charles—given for many saints including the great twelfth-century Crusader noted for his services to the poor—has the common variations of Carl, Carlos, Carlton, Carolo, Carolus, Charley, Charlton and Karl. To honor the Blessed Mother, you might give the name Mary to your daughter—or the name May, Malkin, Maria, Marion, Marianna, Marianne, Marie, Mariette, Marylin, Marian, Maris, Miriam, Marr, Maureen, Maryath, Mae, Molly, Murchie or Murrock. Many other names are associated with the birth, life and sufferings of Our Lady: Alma, Assunta, Carmen, Dolores, Letitia, Mercedes, Pilar, Sharon, Virginia.

His name can have a great meaning for your child. For instance, the name Albert comes from the old Teuton tongue and means "noble and brilliant." A child who has this name and who knows its meaning will be inspired to live up to the ideals it implies.

The saint himself who bore the name will provide inspiration. One of the many Saint Alberts was Albert the Great— a brilliant thirteenth-century scholar who taught theology to Saint Thomas Aquinas and who wrote about forty volumes on a wide range of subjects to earn the title, "Doctor of the Church."

The name Alexander comes from the Greek and means "a helper of mankind." A boy with this name may frequently be reminded that he will achieve a greater success in life if he dedicates himself to serving others, rather than working solely for his own benefit. The name Boniface, from the Latin, means "doer of good." Dominic means "belonging to the Lord." John means "God is gracious." As we learned in studying the New Testament, when Our Lord meant to establish His Church, He mentioned that St. Peter's name meant "rock,"—the rock upon which Jesus wished to build.

Most girls' names also have inspiring meanings. Adelaide, from the Teutonic, means "noble, and of good cheer." Agnes, from the Greek, means "pure, gentle and meek." Angelina, from the Greek, means "angelic." Augusta, from the Latin, means "the exalted." Beatrice is "one who makes happy." Bertha is "bright or glorious." Catherine is "pure," Clare "bright or illustrious," Cordella "warmhearted" and Dorothy "the divine gift."

Preparing for the Baptism service. You need not attend the Baptism service unless you feel well enough to do so. It is customary for the father and godparents to take the infant to church for the ceremony. Some people have a huge celebration on this occasion, but you should not feel obligated to play the hostess unless you are absolutely well. If a family celebration over the baby's birth seems necessary and your economic conditions are such that you would have to do a great deal of work in preparing for it, you should probably defer the party until you are well able to cope with all the demands made upon you.

Nor should you go to needless expense in dressing your baby for his Baptism. If convenient, clothe him in a white robe which has a loose-fitting neckline or can be opened easily at the neck, so that the priest can anoint it with holy oils. White is the preferred color because it symbolizes the purity of soul which will be his after the sacrament is administered. Of course, his Baptism will be valid regardless of how he is dressed.

Your husband or the godparents should be ready to provide the priest with the following information, which will be needed for the church registry: your baby's full name, your home address, father's name, mother's maiden name, name and address of the church in which they were married, when and where the baby was born, and the names of the godparents.

It is customary to make an offering of a few dollars to the priest for performing the ceremony, but this offering is not compulsory. In America, the father generally makes the offering, although in European and Latin-American countries, the godparents frequently do so. If the father makes the offering, the godparents generally give the baby a gift, such as a statue, crucifix, or religious picture, which symbolizes their spiritual relationship.

2

Your Care in Pregnancy

ROBERT J. WALSH, M.D.
Assistant Attending Obstetrician and Gynecologist
St. Vincent's Hospital, New York
Fellow of the American College of Obstetrics and Gynecology

YOU'RE ABOUT TO BECOME A MOTHER

Of course you want the best possible care during your pregnancy to prepare yourself properly for the monumental event that will reach its climax when your baby is born. You want to acquire attitudes and knowledge that will enable you to do a confident and competent job when you return with your newborn from the hospital and set up your home again.

A book like this can help you become a successful parent. It can tell you things expectant mothers generally want to know about themselves and about the growth of the new life within them. It can also answer the questions which are often asked by first-time mothers in particular.

But no book can substitite for your own doctor. Only he can examine you thoroughly to determine whether all is well with you and your growing baby. Only he can prescribe the kind of diet and amount of rest and exercise that may be necessary in your particular case. Only he can answer special questions you may raise or relieve doubts that you may have. And of course only he can be present at your delivery to help you give birth to your baby with a minimum of difficulty. This book can merely strive to help you by describing in general the procedures which usually apply to all births.

Let us start with the beginning of your experience in motherhood—your discovery that you are pregnant. Then we shall review what your pregnancy means to you and your unborn child. We shall consider how you might choose a doctor and hospital, steps you should take at various stages of your pregnancy to insure good health for yourself and your child, common precautions you should follow, danger signals that should put you on your guard, the signs that labor is beginning, and the actual process of birth by which you become the mother of another human being.

How you can tell if you are pregnant. As you doubtless know, the first indication of pregnancy is that you have passed the time of your normally expected menstrual period. The reason is that since you became a woman, your body has constantly maintained a state of readiness for the job of motherhood. It does this by establishing a lining in the uterus each month to nourish the female ovum if it has been fertilized by a male sperm. If there has been such a union, resulting in the creation of a new life, the lining remains as a means of providing the fertilized egg with the nourishment it needs to thrive. If conception does not occur, the lining is disposed of through menstruation, about fourteen days later. Therefore your failure to menstruate may be the first indication that you are pregnant.

There are several other common signs which women observe early in their pregnancy. The breasts may begin to enlarge, the nipples darken, and the entire area becomes more sensitive to touch. You may notice a difference in the amount of saliva you produce, and foods may begin to taste somewhat different. You may find it necessary to urinate more frequently. You may tire more easily or seem to be more nervous. Little things you might have laughed off a few months ago may now upset you.

You may notice mild changes in your gastrointestinal system. Perhaps you feel a twinge of nausea in the morning before you have breakfast, immediately before meals, or when you are very tired.

It is not advisable to wait until all these signs have developed before consulting a physician. He should examine you early in your pregnancy and set up a program to help you pass through the entire period with a minimum of complications. Moreover, it is important to have someone who knows your record whom you could call immediately should an unexpected development occur. As a general rule, you should visit a physician if you miss two menstrual periods. This would be about six weeks after conception has taken place.

Choosing your doctor. You will obtain the best treatment during your pregnancy if you consult an obstetrician—a doctor who specializes in the care of pregnant women, who has had special training in meeting any problems encountered during pregnancy, and who is familiar with the new medicines and methods of treatment constantly being developed to make childbirth safer.

You can obtain the name of a qualified obstetrician by asking your family doctor to recommend one. Or you might call the County or State Medical Society, or a recognized hospital in your community in which obstetrical cases are handled, asking them for a list of doctors who specialize in this practice. If an obstetrician is on the staff of a hospital which has a good record, you can be confident that he is qualified. Your pastor usually can recommend a qualified obstetrician-gynecologist through his contacts in parish work. You may also obtain the name of a competent obstetrician in your area by writing for this information to the American College of Obstetricians and Gynecologists, 79 West Monroe Street, Chicago 3, Illinois.

Obstetricians can now be found in almost all medium-sized

and large communities throughout the country. Thanks to the automobile and the telephone, you can receive this expert medical care almost anywhere. In the open West, for example, women often drive fifty miles within an hour for their monthly medical examination, and can phone the doctor at any time in an emergency.

If you cannot avail yourself of an obstetrician's services, consult your family doctor. He will either take you under his personal care or suggest where more specialized treatment and supervision are obtainable. Family doctors have delivered millions of babies with safety, of course, and they are usually conscientious in referring their patients to a specialist if a situation arises with which they have had little experience. In this day and age there is no excuse for women to put themselves in the hands of midwives equipped neither by training nor intellect to handle even routine deliveries. It is a fact that most deaths associated with pregnancy occur when expectant mothers fail to avail themselves of the best medical service in their communities.

Your first visit to the obstetrician. This will be a "get acquainted" session. You should feel free to ask any questions concerning fees, treatments, possible complications or difficulties you anticipate. Your doctor will treat the entire discussion in confidence.

He or his nurse will ask a number of questions about your background. Your answers will often give him valuable clues about your physical condition and may indicate to him what special treatments may be required. You will be asked about illnesses you may have had, about your parents, whether you have been pregnant before and had a successful delivery, and similar questions. Your replies will be carefully recorded to give him a permanent file he can use in setting up a routine for you to follow. He will add to his records each time you visit him, and thus will always have an up-to-date chart of your condition.

At your first visit, he may want to examine you completely, or may do only a pelvic examination, depending on whether he is pressed for time at that moment. His nurse will ask you to disrobe in the dressing room, and you will be given a gown to cover yourself.

You must understand that an obstetrician's time is not his own, and he may be late for office appointments, or may have to leave during office hours to care for someone about to deliver.

When you arranged for your first visit, you may have been asked to bring a specimen of your urine with you, or you may now be asked to pass urine into a container in the doctor's office. This urine provides valuable clues about your physical condition. For example, if it contains sugar, it may indicate that you have a diabetic condition and thus will require special care.

Another test can be done to determine whether you are actually pregnant. A small amount of your urine or blood can be sent to a laboratory, where it will be injected into a test animal—usually a rat or a rabbit or a mouse. A chemical substance in the urine and blood of a pregnant woman causes almost immediate changes in the reproductive organs of these animals. Therefore these changes are virtually certain evidence that you are pregnant. Such a test may be done early in pregnancy—perhaps soon after the first menstrual period is missed —and is especially valuable if the state of the prospective mother's health requires that a special routine be established at once. This test costs about ten dollars. In the average case, no pregnancy test is needed.

After you have missed two periods, an obstetrician can usually determine by pelvic examination whether you are pregnant or not. Usually, there is much undue apprehension concerning the pelvic examination, because for most patients this is the first time they have been examined vaginally. With gentleness and reassurance the patient relaxes, and the examination is completed without the discomfort that was feared. Using a small light, the obstetrician can inspect the vagina, and can see the mouth of the uterus, which is called the cervix. With one or two fingers, he can feel the uterus and tell by its size and shape if there is any enlargement. When an enlarged uterus is coupled with other signs—skipped menstrual period, changes in your breasts, etc.—the evidence of pregnancy is fairly conclusive.

The doctor will go on to a more detailed examination of your head and neck, heart, lungs, breasts and abdomen. Your blood pressure will be taken. He will also take a sample of your blood by pricking your arm with a small needle to which a tube is attached. He will take little more than a spoonful, yet this amount will enable a laboratory to tell him many important things about you. For example: The blood count will tell if you are anemic—a condition usually due to a lack of iron—and thus will need a higher intake of iron in food and by tablets to bring it up to normal. It will determine whether you have an infection—indicated by an excess of white blood cells—which must be cleared up. And it will establish whether you are Rh-positive or Rh-negative, as well as your blood type. A test for syphilis is also required by law.

While the doctor must await laboratory reports to complete the picture of your condition, he will be able, in almost all cases, to tell whether you are pregnant. He will also be able to approximate when the baby will be born. You can make this estimate yourself. The birth date is generally about 280 days from the 1st day of the last menstrual period, or 266 days from the day of conception, if this is known. To determine the date, recall the first day of your last period. Then go back to the same date three months previously and add seven days. Suppose that your last menstrual period began August 9. You would go back three months to May 9. By adding seven days, you would arrive at May 16 as the expected date of your baby's birth.

Of course, some babies are born weeks before the anticipated date, and others are not delivered until several weeks after it. However, most babies are born within a week on either side of the date arrived at by the formula above.

During the interview, your doctor will outline steps you should take to get adequate diet, rest and exercise. If you are overweight, he will suggest special foods to help you reduce so that you will have a more comfortable pregnancy. If you are underweight, he may suggest a diet which contains more calories than are necessary for your daily needs. The extra calories are then converted into body fat.

He will also tell you how often he expects to see you during your pregnancy. Patients usually have a checkup every month until the sixth or seventh month, and then see the doctor more frequently until the last month, when they often make weekly visits.

If your obstetrician delivers babies at more than one hospital, you may be given an option of choosing the hospital and the type of care (private or semiprivate) you wish to receive. If you select your obstetrician carefully, you can be confident that the hospitals at which he practices are equally reputable. In any event, the hospital should be accredited by the American Hospital Association, should have the endorsement of the local medical society, and should enjoy a good reputation in the community. If you are in doubt, ask your family doctor or another physician in whom you have confidence, your local Public Health nurse, or your local medical society.

Feel free to discuss fees. Most obstetricians charge a flat sum for all their services during pregnancy. This includes regular examinations and care during pregnancy, delivery of the baby in the hospital, care of the mother in the hospital after delivery, and a final checkup after she returns home. Because of this custom, the woman who delays visiting an obstetrician actually saves no money and fails to obtain advice and aid which would be hers at no additional cost. This is especially true of the post partum examination which is so important and often neglected.

If you are unable to pay his fee, you should tell him so *now*. He may be able to make an adjustment, or to suggest an install- ment method of payment which will be easier on you. (Many couples today prefer the "pay as you go" system so that the hos- pital bill and the doctor's bill are not both due at the same time.) If you know that you cannot pay the fee, he probably can help you obtain care within your income level.

Be sure to mention the fact if you have medical or hospital insurance. Many obstetricians join Blue Shield or other plans by which the insurance company pays a part of their fee. How- ever, you will find that maternity allowances, in general, are poor, compared to other types of surgical allowances. Therefore it will pay you to read your policies carefully to avoid future disappointments.

If you took out a policy at a specified time, usually at least ten months before you became pregnant, the insurance com- pany will allow a small set amount toward your hospital bill, whether you choose a semiprivate or private room, and you must pay the difference. Some obstetricians charge one fee for patients who take private rooms and a lesser fee for those who take semiprivate accommodations. Some think there is little jus- tification for this, since some wealthy patients like company, and some poorer patients like or require privacy. When compli- cations arise, the fee is usually higher. Your doctor will explain these factors if you ask him about them.

Does your doctor inspire your confidence? During your first visit, you will have an opportunity to form an opinion about the obstetrician, perhaps to decide that his personality puts you at ease, that his approach in no way violates your sense of mod- esty, and that his general manner is competent and reassuring and inspires confidence. Your relationship with him will be very personal, and you should feel free to choose a doctor in whom you can confide your deepest thoughts and receive sympathetic consideration for your innermost fears. This first interview works both ways and unless the obstetrician feels that he can work with you, he may suggest that you seek help from someone else.

It is especially important, of course, that he be one who will respect your religious and moral convictions. In normal pregnancies moral questions usually do not arise. Sometimes, however, suggestions are made that the patient submit to practices opposed to the moral law—that she have a "therapeutic" abortion, submit to sterilization to prevent future pregnancies, or practice methods of artificial birth control which violate her religious convictions. If your doctor knows that you are a Catholic, and you should so inform him, he probably will not make suggestions which run counter to your moral codes. If he persists in suggesting such procedures, you are perfectly within your rights in choosing another physician. But this step is rarely necessary with a man who is experienced with the moral teachings of the Church as they apply to obstetrical and gynecological problems.

If all goes well during your first visit, you will leave your doctor's office with your expectation of motherhood confirmed. You will know that you are in good hands and have excellent prospects of giving birth to a normal baby if you follow the program he has outlined. You should also feel that he will be able to help you with any phsyical or emotional problems which might arise. In brief, after this initial visit, you should feel that you have an adviser in whom you can place full confidence.

Statistics prove childbirth is safe. If you consult an obstetrician when you have good evidence that you are pregnant, and if you make plans early to have your baby in a reputable hospital, you will provide the best possible assurance that you will carry your baby to full term and that both of you will survive in good health.

Medical advances in the past quarter-century have taken most of the risks out of childbearing. Figures compiled by the National Office of Vital Statistics prove this point. In 1930, when many of the present readers were born, one mother died for each 150 live births in the United States.

In 1950, there was one maternal death in 1,200 live births. Today, the maternal death rate has dropped another 55 per cent since 1950, so that now only one mother is lost for every 2,500 babies born alive. So we see that the rate of maternal mortality today has been reduced tremendously from what it was in 1930. It is therefore quite obvious that your chances of coming through pregnancy today are far greater than they were in your mother's day.

Furthermore, these figures tell only part of the story, for they include the rate for areas where many babies are born at home and delivered by midwives. If we excluded those who cannot or will not take advantage of modern obstetrical care and the facilities of modern hospitals, the rate would be even lower. For example, in eight states where almost all women have their babies in hospitals under good medical care, the rate is less than three deaths for every 10,000 live births.

These figures are worth considering because some young women still regard childbearing as both difficult and dangerous. Undeniably, it was so at one time. Possibly you have heard stories from your mother or grandmother about the hazards associated with giving birth. But, as the statistics prove, this experience is no longer one that you should dread.

The truly spectacular reductions in both maternal and infant mortality in recent times results from many factors. One of the most important is that the modern woman places herself under an obstetrician's care early in her pregnancy. Another is her recognition that if she cooperates, modern medicine can ease her pregnancy and make it as painless as it has ever been in history.

The modern emphasis on maintaining a good figure means a great deal also. As we shall see, obesity is one of the hazards that you must guard against as your pregnancy progresses. If you keep your weight down, you will maintain your own vitality and energy and you will deliver your baby more easily. You may be excused some stoutness while carrying your baby, but you will be called to account after birth. Then you will want to regain your slender figure and slip easily into dresses you had laid aside for the duration.

The main reason childbirth has become so safe, however, has been that we now can virtually chart the progress of the pregnancy. By routine periodic visits, we can accurately record the growth and position of the baby at various stages of its development. Through blood tests, urine analyses, tests of blood pressure and the like, we can maintain a close check on the physical condition of the mother and treat any conditions which might cause trouble later. We now have a better knowledge of the important part that good nutrition plays in strengthening the mother and in giving the fetus all the necessary nutrients for good health and vitality. We have made spectacular progress in treating diseases which were once dangerous for both mother and child. We have better drugs to prevent infection or its spread. Improved anesthetics and improved ways of administering them, and improved operating room procedures and surgical equipment, all add to the present-day safety of childbirth.

As a result of these and other factors, years intervene between cases of a mother dying in childbirth in a modern hospital. Cases that do occur are usually the result of the expectant mother's indifference, of her ignorance or unwillingness to consult a doctor early in pregnancy, or of her failure to follow his suggestions or report changes in her condition while he might still treat them effectively.

As an expectant mother, you can be reassured by the fact

that the modern obstetrician and modern hospital have the knowledge and equipment to make your experience safe and trouble-free. You can assure yourself of a successful pregnancy if you carefully follow the program of diet, rest and exercise which your doctor prescribes, if you keep alert to changes in your condition which should be reported to him immediately, and if you develop the calm, cheerful attitude about your pregnancy which is fully warranted by the facts.

THE STORY OF YOUR PREGNANCY

It will help you to understand why certain steps are necessary in your pregnancy if you have a general knowledge of how your baby was conceived, how he draws nourishment from you as he develops within your womb, and the process by which he finally leaves your body and begins his life independently of you. This is a remarkable story in which you should feel honored to play the important role. For no matter how often the miracles of conception and birth may be repeated, they remain eternally exciting and awe-inspiring.

How conception occurs. In intercourse, about three hundred million sperm are deposited into the vagina. In order that conception take place, one sperm must penetrate an egg usually in the Fallopian tube. This fertilized egg then travels to the uterus, where it will remain and grow until the baby is born.

As you probably know, an egg is released from one of the two ovaries in a woman's body approximately every 28 days. If there is no fertilization by the sperm, there is no conception. The lining in the uterus, prepared to provide nourishment to the new being, is then disposed of through menstruation.

If conception has occurred, however, the fertilized egg will pass into the uterus and will begin to draw nourishment from it. The one cell will divide into two and the two into four in a process of multiplication and differentiation until the baby, made up of millions of such tiny cells, finally leaves the womb.

As this tiny cell enters the uterus, it already contains much of the baby's inheritance. A miracle in itself is the fact that in this tiny fertilized egg—which can hardly be seen by the un-aided eye—are factors which will determine your child's physical appearance, some of his mental abilities and such talents as an aptitude for music or art. In that fused ovum, the blood type, the color of the eyes and skin, the shape of some of the facial features and the sex have already been determined.

Parents of large families are often amazed to discover that one child is so unlike another. Children may differ not only in appearance, but also in personality, talents and intelligence. But this is a matter over which you have little control. If you can understand this fact, you will realize that your child has a God-given personality of his own—one which you can mold so as to make him a responsible, respectable adult, but which you will be unable to change completely.

How the new life feeds and grows. The male sperm usually unites with the ovum in one of the two Fallopian tubes. These tubes are about three inches long and one-sixth inch in diameter, and lie between the uterus and the ovary. After about three days, the fertilized egg moves into the uterus. At first, the new life gets its food from within the egg itself. At the end of six days, it requires another source of food or will die from starvation. It finds this food source in the blood vessels lining the walls of the uterus, and it develops tiny finger-like feelers which attach themselves to the lining and draw nourishment from your blood.

During its first three months of development, the fertilized egg is known as the embryo. As it grows, it continues to send out feelers. Gradually the placenta, a soft, cushiony tissue, develops along the uterine walls. Blood vessels from the embryo reach into the placenta through the umbilical cord, and by this means the embryo draws food from your blood stream and its waste products are carried to your body where you dispose of them in the normal processes of elimination. But no direct connection exists between your blood vessels and those of the embryo.

A thin membrane also develops at the edges of the placenta, and a watery fluid accumulates within it. This membrane encloses the baby's body in a fluid environment. It serves as a cushion, protecting him against bumps that would otherwise occur as your body shifts position in your ordinary activities. In a sense the developing infant remains under water for nine months. How is this possible? The answer, of course, is that at this stage he does not need air to breathe as he will after birth. Instead, he draws the necessary oxygen for his life processes from your blood stream. His lungs will not be used to inhale and exhale air until he leaves your body.

During the first three months of pregnancy, the embryo will continue to strengthen its hold upon the walls of the uterus. Once established, it grows with increasing rapidity. Two weeks after conception, it would be possible to see its outline with your naked eye. After one month, it is about one-sixth of an inch long and the head is much larger, proportionately, than the rest of the body.

Now the vital organs—heart, liver, brain, lungs—begin to form. Within another two weeks the backbone will begin to develop, and tiny limbs—later to become legs and arms—will start to grow out from the body.

About the twelfth week of pregnancy, a significant milestone is passed. Now the placenta and membranes probably are firmly in place. The body is perhaps as much as three inches long and has begun to take a human shape we can recognize. The arms and legs are more fully developed. As though to mark this progress, the little body is from now on until birth referred to as the fetus.

You are now inescapably aware of the fact that you are pregnant. Even if you did not observe any of the usual signs before, they are unavoidable by this time. Your abdomen is growing. Your breasts are becoming larger, preparing for the natural act of feeding your baby after he is born. The nipples are distinctly darker.

You begin to "feel life." Another great milestone will occur about the twentieth week—the end of the fifth lunar month. The fetus will be about nine inches long. It will weigh from eight to twelve ounces, and its outline will show unmistakable human qualities. The facial features will be well formed, the arms and legs will be almost full-sized in proportion to the rest of the body, and the internal organs will be large and well developed.

The heartbeat now is stronger, and it may be heard by the doctor for the first time. Probably you will also feel movement or "life," as the fetus moves about. At first you may think it is "gas," but as it persists and becomes stronger you come to realize there is an active baby within your own body and for the first time truly recognize the great gift which God has given you. From now on, fetal movements will become more and more obvious and quite often there seems to be more activity at night.

By now, you will probably weigh five to eight pounds over your usual weight. You will have to store away the slips and dresses you wore before you became pregnant, and content yourself with clothing that fits loosely over your body. Because of your changing body physiology, you may tire more easily and may find it necessary to take more frequent naps. It may be more difficult for you to climb stairs, to remain on your feet for long periods, or to get by on the same amount of sleep you were accustomed to before conception. This is a normal protective mechanism.

What happens during the last stage of pregnancy. At the end of twenty-eight weeks, or seven lunar months, you begin the third and final trimester. By now, all of your baby's organs have been developed. His shape is like that of a baby at full term. If an accident should now occur and the baby were born prematurely in a hospital where special facilities were available, the chances for survival would be good. Of course, the development he will undergo in your womb in the final period will give him a better start in life, for there is no incubator as good as your own uterus.

In these last weeks, the baby gains strength and puts on a layer of fat. By the time he reaches full term, his facial features may be sharp and clearly defined. He will have a fuzzy beginning of hair on his head. His skin will be firm and clear and close to its normal color.

If he is average, he will weigh about seven to seven and a half pounds and will be about twenty inches long. It is desirable that he be neither too small nor too large. Some babies are more than two feet long and weigh fifteen pounds or more. Of course, it is a great deal more difficult for the mother to carry and give birth to such a child.

During labor, the water sac surrounding the baby may break or the doctor may break the sac artificially, to improve the quality of labor and thus implement the delivery of the baby through the birth canal.

When the baby has emerged, the doctor will tie the umbilical cord and divide it and then the baby is on his own, your body having completed its role in bringing forth new life. The placenta will separate and pass out through the birth canal in the normal third stage of labor and your pregnancy will be concluded.

A PROGRAM FOR PREGNANCY

Your doctor will give you specific advice on what you should eat and when, on drinking and smoking, exercise, sexual activity, and on many other subjects during the various stages of pregnancy. His is the advice to follow, because he gives it with a personal knowledge of your case.

However, there are many suggestions which are given to almost all expectant mothers. And when your doctor outlines a procedure for you to follow, this is the kind of advice he is likely to give:

Foods to eat and to avoid. You will need a balance of vitamins, minerals, proteins, carbohydrates and fats, because the food you eat must nourish not only your own body but that of your child. You should eat foods which are high in protein (or body-building) value and high in vitamin and mineral content, and avoid foods high in calories which may provide energy but only add weight when consumed in excess quantities.

You should take special care to avoid putting on extra weight. If you gain too much, you will be uncomfortable during the middle and later stages of your pregnancy. You will be unable to move around as easily as you might do otherwise, and you may be unable to remain active even for relatively short periods without feeling tired. However, there does not seem to be any scientific support for the old opinion that if you gain too much weight, your baby also may gain too much.

Your diet will also be important later if you plan to nurse your baby. Good dietary habits established during the pregnancy are easy to continue afterwards to insure adequate nutritional advantages of your own milk.

In order to get all the proteins you will need, your diet should contain plenty of milk (as much as a quart every day) along with other dairy products like cheese. You should have at least one serving of meat, poultry or fish every day, an average of perhaps one egg a day. Especially valuable are meats such as liver which have a high iron content and help to combat anemia.

You will get some vitamins and minerals from the above foods. You should also have at least one large serving per day of citrus fruits or tomatoes—which are rich in vitamin C—and another large serving of dark-green or deep-yellow vegetables for their vitamin A. Bread or cereals you eat should be of the whole grain, enriched or restored type because they have more vitamin B and iron than the ordinary kind.

Eat less of other foods—especially pastries, fatty foods, sweet desserts—which supply relatively little nourishment but have a high caloric content. Drink four to six glasses of water a day plus the milk, in order to provide enough fluids for good kidney functioning. Have at least one daily serving of a raw fruit or vegetable—perhaps an apple, a lettuce salad or raw carrot sticks —because they help regulate your bowel movements as well as providing a good source of vitamins.

Modern doctors prescribe vitamin and mineral supplements as a matter of course, since it has been shown that the average patient needs them because of the increased requirements in pregnancy.

An old wives' tale holds that every baby costs his mother a tooth. This belief probably originated because extra amounts of calcium are needed to build bone structure and teeth, and the fetus draws calcium from the mother during pregnancy. Today there is no need to "lose a tooth for a child." In addition to recommending milk, custards, puddings or sherbert—all rich in calcium—your doctor will prescribe tablets which also contain the mineral in concentrated form.

As your special needs require, he may make other suggestions. For instance, to prevent retention of body water, he may want you to eliminate or reduce salty foods—ham and bacon, salted peanuts, potato chips and the like. You can get accustomed to food cooked without salt more easily than you think. Your husband need not make the sacrifice with you. He can add salt to his food after it is on the table. You may add extra flavor to your food by adding pepper or lemon juice.

How to control your weight. Naturally, you will gain weight during pregnancy. If your baby is average, he will weigh about seven to seven and a half pounds. The placenta and amniotic fluid will weigh about three pounds, and your enlarged uterus and breasts about three and a half pounds, meaning that the total extra weight will amount to about fourteen pounds. In addition, you will have a normal tendency to retain more water in your body.

As a result of these factors, many doctors seek to prevent a weight gain of more than fifteen pounds in patients who are of average weight to begin with. This means that in the last thirty weeks of pregnancy—when most of the weight is added —you will be "on target" if you gain no more than half a pound a week.

Keeping well and comfortable. Another important factor that will contribute to both your physical and emotional well-being is adequate exercise. You will probably be permitted to continue most of the activities in which you normally engage, if no complicating factors are present. If you play tennis, ride horses or indulge in other strenuous sports, you will probably have to curtail them until your baby is born.

Sports in which you might be permitted to indulge moderately are golf, bathing and swimming—the latter provided that the water is calm and not too cold. Diving and prolonged swimming generally are frowned upon at this time.

You may be allowed to drive an automobile up to the final stages, when your baby might come between you and the steering wheel anyway. But avoid extensive driving over bumpy roads and driving for long distances without relief. If you must drive a long distance, choose well-paved roads, if possible, and spend no more than ninety minutes in the car at one time. Break up the trip with rest periods of fifteen minutes or longer during which you get out and walk about. Long railroad, airplane or sea trips might also be avoided. Before taking one, consult your doctor. You will probably be told to curtail strenuous housework like scrubbing floors or carrying heavy baskets of wet clothing from your washing machine to your drying yard. But you probably will be permitted to continue routine activities—preparing meals and cleaning up after them, vacuuming and dusting, doing light gardening and the like.

Try to spend time in the open air every day. If you can, stroll to the nearby shops or park, following a route where you can sit and relax a while in the open if you become tired. You might carry light purchases—a loaf of bread, a quart of milk, etc.—back from the store with you, but it might be better to drive your car or bring along a cart if you have a large number of items to carry.

Spending a few hours out of doors each day will accomplish several important purposes. The sun and air serve as a general tonic for the body, and mild exercise will help your circulation and digestion, help your body eliminate waste matter, and help you to relax.

Also try to get fresh air at night. Even in cold weather, sleep with the windows open at least slightly. If you can, avoid smoke-filled rooms and keep fresh air circulating in rooms where you spend a great deal of time.

Adequate sleep and rest are essential. You need eight hours of uninterrupted sleep at night, plus frequent rest periods and a nap during the day. If you are doing housework, try to get off your feet occasionally and do some jobs in a resting or reclining position. Try to take a nap regularly. After lunch or in the late afternoon are times that many women find conducive to a short sleep.

Precautions for working women. Some states have enacted special regulations covering the conditions under which expectant mothers may work outside their homes. Many industries themselves have set up standards to minimize the risk that any tasks assigned a pregnant woman will endanger her health or that of the fetus.

Special safeguards may be necessary for those in jobs which require a great deal of standing, moving about, or other physical activity. You might ask your employer to transfer you to a job which will enable you to sit down, or to get off your feet at frequent intervals. Some tasks which are ordinarily performed standing up can be done just as well by a person seated upon a high stool. Office workers, cashiers, shop clerks, etc., probably can get off their feet often enough during the day so as to eliminate any problems in that respect.

When should you stop working? A job requiring much physical activity—constant standing or much lifting or bending, for example—should not be continued after the fifth month. If you have a job you can perform almost entirely in a sitting position, and also have facilities where you can occasionally lie down during the day, there probably is no physical reason why you could not continue it until the last month.

The employment question is one you should discuss with your doctor. He can tell from your physical condition, the nature of your work, and your progress in pregnancy, whether and when discontinuing your job would be advisable.

Dress for comfort. Your pregnancy will be somewhat less complicated if you make up your mind to dress primarily for comfort during this period. This does not mean that you should disregard style entirely. In fact, dress manufacturers have made great strides in recent years in creating garments for pregnant women that are both attractive and serviceable. But if you must choose between comfort and chic, you might be well advised to choose the former and console yourself with the thought that you will again be stylish after you give birth.

You probably need not wear maternity garments until after the fourth month. After that time, you should wear underclothing, slips, skirts and dresses that will neither fit tightly nor put too much pressure upon your waistline.

Dresses, skirts and slips should rest upon the shoulders and should have adequate width around the midsection. They will then hang loosely and put no weight or pressure upon the abdomen. Avoid tight-fitting garments, such as knitted sweaters.

You will probably find it necessary to wear a larger brassiere. One which lifts each breast up and inward, toward the opposite shoulder, and which has a wide, sturdy shoulder strap is often recommended.

You may need a special abdominal support after the third or fourth month of pregnancy. An ordinary girdle or corset will not be suitable because of its limited stretching potential. A maternity girdle has sides and back you can tie with straps. These can be loosened as your uterus expands. Your doctor will advise you if this extra support seems to be necessary. Maternity corsets are stocked by most shops which specialize in apparel for expectant mothers. The important thing to remember about abdominal supports is to pull them on while lying down, so that when you get up, they support instead of crush you.

You will have to do without round garters for the duration. They tend to hamper the circulation of blood in the legs and might contribute to varicose veins or cramps in the leg muscles. You may find it comfortable to do without stockings and wear ankle socks most of the time. When you dress up, you might use a garter belt supported from the shoulders, rather than the abdomen. Many women have reported that these belts are reasonably comfortable and satisfactory.

High-heeled shoes or "spikes" should also be avoided. They tend to throw your body off balance and as your weight increases, you will find it increasingly difficult to support yourself upon them. But you need not go the extreme of wearing shoes with almost no heel. A good compromise which combines comfort with safety is a broader heel of medium height—one perhaps half as high as the shoes you usually wear. You will also find these shoes useful after the baby is born.

Smoking and drinking—how much is permitted? Some research indicates that when a mother inhales cigarette smoke, a temporary increase can be noted in the heartbeat of the fetus. However, there is no evidence to support the belief that smoking in moderation will endanger your child's development. Many doctors consider smoking "moderate" when less than twenty cigarettes are consumed in a twenty-four-hour period. Recent reports show that babies of smoking mothers tend to be smaller than those of nonsmokers.

What you should do about smoking will depend, of course, upon your doctor's judgment of your own particular case. Smoking may tend to aggravate such conditions as high blood pressure and nervous tension. Perhaps you will be told to restrict your intake of nicotine in order to prevent other difficulties in pregnancy.

The "rule of moderation" also applies to drinking. One cocktail or highball or a glass of wine or beer usually is thought to be harmless for the average expectant mother. In fact, a drink before dinner or in the evening may help you relax—an important aid at this time. But drinking to excess is dangerous, not only because it disturbs your bodily functions but because it increases the danger of falls or accidents which might cause complications. Many women find that they "can't stand" alcohol during pregnancy, and some find this the earliest sign of pregnancy.

Care of the skin and breasts. Since you will now discharge your baby's wastes as well as your own, your organs of excretion will have more work to do. Your skin is an important means by which you discharge waste matter through perspiration.

During pregnancy, you are likely to perspire more than at other times. There may be a tendency for odors to develop. To keep your skin in good condition, you should wash your body every day—preferably by taking a shower. Dry yourself by rubbing a towel briskly all over your body. Hot baths should be avoided, and tub baths should be avoided as you get larger and tend to lose your balance more easily, in order to prevent slipping and possible injury getting in and out of the tub.

A shower will therefore be safer in the final months of pregnancy. The shower area should have a support, solidly attached to the wall, which you can hold while washing yourself.

After the fourth month or so, you may have to pay special attention to your breasts and nipples. Around that time a colorless secretion may begin to come from the nipples. This is a step in preparing your breasts for the act of feeding your baby. Be sure to wash the nipples with a soft cloth and mild soap and water. Sometimes the secretion will harden and a slight scaling will remain attached to the nipples. It will generally come off if you gently apply a little cold cream at night, leave it on until morning, and then wash with soap and water.

In order to prepare the nipples for nursing, some doctors suggest the regular application of cocoa butter during the last weeks of pregnancy. However, do not undertake any "do-it-yourself" treatment without the approval of your own doctor. Today, most doctors feel that no nipple preparation is necessary and that it may do more harm than good.

Care of the teeth. As noted previously, there is now no reason to believe that "every child must cost a tooth." But dental care during pregnancy is important. If neglected, infected teeth or gums may affect your whole body.

If you have not visited your dentist within six months, see him soon after you know you are pregnant, and obtain a thorough checkup. He should fill any cavities and treat any infected teeth. You will find it easier to complete the work now, because you will find little time after the baby arrives. Contrary to some old beliefs, you run no danger of miscarriage in having necessary dental work done during pregnancy. Nor is there any truth to the superstition that your baby will be harmed in some way if one of your teeth is pulled at this time.

Brush your teeth regularly after every meal if possible, and use an astringent mouth wash if your gums have a tendency to bleed.

Intercourse during pregnancy. Many ancient peoples believed it dangerous to engage in sexual relations during pregnancy, and they practiced strict abstinence at this time. Some researchers trace the practice of polygamy—one man having many wives—to the primitive male's desire to circumvent this custom. On the other hand, ancient Greeks thought frequent intercourse helpful to the health of both mother and fetus. Other ancients regarded it as dangerous during the first and last trimesters of pregnancy, but relatively harmless during the middle period.

Even today, doctors do not fully agree. This is so partly because each woman's constitution must be considered individually; what may be suitable for one may be undesirable for another.

The advice generally given, however, is that you should omit intercourse on the days you would have had your second and third menstrual periods had you not become pregnant. At this time, some pregnant women experience slight cramps—a faint relative of menstrual cramps—and it is thought that excessive agitation might induce miscarriage.

Under ordinary circumstances, your doctor may say that intercourse is permissible in moderation until about six weeks before the baby is due. Marital relations during the last six weeks are advised against because of the danger that premature labor might ensue.

Some women notice a change in their attitude regarding intercourse during pregnancy, as well as a change in the way they respond to their husband's advances. Some experience a greater intensity of desire than ever before. Others lose all interest in sex and remain unmoved by stimuli to which they formerly responded. There is no reason to become concerned in either event. If you are considerate of your husband's needs and desires—and he is considerate of yours—an adjustment during this temporary period can doubtless be made. On this matter— and in the others outlined in this chapter—your doctor will be your best adviser.

NORMAL PROBLEMS YOU MAY ENCOUNTER

You can expect a certain number of physical discomforts as your baby develops within you. Some result from your condition itself. Others, which may occur occasionally at other times, now may be more conspicuous. These discomforts include:

Constipation. This condition is fairly common in pregnancy, and results from the general sluggishness of the bowels caused by the changes due to the pregnancy itself. Even the most "regular" women may become constipated in pregnancy. This can usually be overcome by dietary changes. It may also become more evident if you fail to take regular exercise or drink enough liquids.

The establishment of regular bowel habits is a good way to prevent constipation or to keep it from becoming habitual. Try to move your bowels at the same time each day—preferably during a regular period when you can relax. Like many others, you may find that this period occurs in the morning, after your husband has left for work and before you begin your daily housekeeping routine. Fruits and vegetables are good aids to body regularity. Try to eat five or six servings of vegetables or fruits each day, including a leafy green or deep-yellow vegetable and a raw vegetable and fruit. They will supply the roughage to produce a well-formed stool. Some mothers find that a glass of water just before bedtime and a glass of water or fruit juice the first thing in the morning also are helpful.

If natural methods of dealing with constipation do not achieve results, consult your doctor. Never dose yourself with laxatives or take enemas without his explicit instructions.

More frequent urination. During the early months of pregnancy, most women complain that they urinate more often than usual, and they also report this condition during the final weeks. The condition results from the fact that the bladder is located just in front of the uterus. As the uterus expands, it exerts pressure on the lower part of the bladder, creating the urge to urinate more frequently. During the middle period of pregnancy, the baby's position is changed and the pressure is relieved. Along about the eighth month, the position changes again and the baby begins to move downwards. Now the pressure may even create a tendency to pass slight amounts of urine involuntarily. For example, there may be a slight leakage if you cough or laugh heartily.

You should not find this condition annoying if you recognize that it will end when your pregnancy ends. If the need to urinate interrupts your sleep, your doctor may urge you not to drink fluids after dinner. You may then dispose of most of the urine in your system before you retire.

Nausea and "morning sickness." Despite what you may have heard, nausea is not necessary. True, many women suffer some degree of it, but others go through the entire nine months without any difficulty. It is more likely to strike a woman with a sensitive digestive system, one who is inclined to worry, or one who finds it difficult to relax.

Understanding and acting upon a simple fact will help relieve nausea. It is that you are more likely to feel it if your stomach is empty. Therefore if you eat a number of small meals throughout the day instead of three large meals, your stomach will always retain some food—and you will feel less disturbed by nausea.

It is important, however, to eat low-calorie foods which will fill you up without increasing your weight excessively. Soda crackers and dry or lightly buttered toast are often recommended.

You might leave a few crackers by your bed at night. On awakening, munch on them to relieve or prevent the "morning sickness" which results from not having eaten any food during the night. If you rest in bed for fifteen or twenty minutes after eating the crackers, you will probably find it easier to get up and about.

For breakfast, try to eat less than you would normally. Fruit juice, cereal with milk or cream, toast and coffee may be suitable. After eating, try to relax a while to aid your digestion before you begin your housework.

Another small snack may be advisable in midmorning—perhaps crackers or dry toast with milk, cocoa or tea. For lunch, you might try a light meal of soup or broth, a vegetable salad or fruit, bread or crackers, and coffee, tea or milk.

Another light snack might be eaten in midafternoon. Your dinner might consist of slightly smaller portions than you might normally take. Before retiring, eat a few crackers—and perhaps a glass of milk.

If you tend to suffer from nausea, eliminate foods that are hard to digest. These include greasy foods like bacon and pork chops, foods fried in fats or oils, and vegetables like cabbage and cauliflower which tend to induce a gaseous condition.

Some women find that drinking water aggravates their condition. If this is true in your case, substitute other liquids—milk, soups, soft drinks made with sugar substitutes which have no caloric value, or cocoa. You might add more coffee or tea to your diet if the extra quantities do not cause sleeplessness at night.

Very sweet foods like cookies and candies do not seem to be very helpful and are high in calories. If you resort to them to appease your gnawing feeling, you may soon find your weight increasing at a dangerous rate.

If nausea persists despite more frequent eating, try to lie down after each meal and to assume as relaxed a position and attitude as possible. At other times, tests have proved that if a person can take her mind off her condition, the sense of nausea will diminish or disappear entirely. So try to read a good, gripping novel. Watch television, if you can find programs that hold your interest. Invite friends to come in and chat. Or figure out other ways to get your mind off your condition for a time.

Three thoughts may make your nausea at least a little more

bearable. First, since it generally is worse in the morning, you might console yourself that things will get better as the day goes on. Secondly, "morning sickness" will generally disappear almost entirely after the third month, when your body has adjusted itself to pregnancy. Finally, you hold it within your own power to relieve your condition—partly, at least—by following proper rules of diet, by relaxing wherever possible, and by turning your mind to other subjects whenever you can. Your doctor can prescribe various new medications which are most helpful for this problem.

Heartburn. Despite its name, this condition is not related to any functioning of the heart. It is so called because it results in a burning sensation high in the stomach, near the heart. It is most likely to occur during the last weeks of pregnancy. It results from the fact that the fetus has now grown so large that it exerts pressure against the stomach, making it more difficult for normal digestive processes to go on. In connection with heartburn, there may be occasional belching and a regurgitation of small amounts of digestive juices.

You can prevent or minimize heartburn by developing eating habits that do not place too great a burden on your digestive processes. It may help to take a small amount of cream about twenty minutes before eating. This helps to stimulate the intestines and to encourage the movement of food through the digestive tract. During the meal proper, however, avoid any rich, greasy, or fried foods which are difficult to digest. Take small portions into your mouth, and chew slowly and thoroughly. Try to make mealtimes as relaxed and pleasant as possible.

Some women gain relief by chewing gum after meals, others by taking a spoonful of milk of magnesia about twenty minutes after each meal and before retiring. Heartburn remedies other than these should not be taken without specific instructions from your doctor. Avoid bicarbonate of soda unless he specifically tells you to use it.

Flatulence. This condition results from the accumulation of gas in the alimentary canal. It is usually characterized by a distention of the intestines. There is often a bloated feeling, and the frequent necessity to pass gas. Sometimes flatulence and heartburn go together. Or gas may exist without heartburn.

If flatulence disturbs you as you advance in pregnancy, you can relieve it by regular evacuation of your bowels, taking a tablespoonful of milk of magnesia after each meal to stimulate the movement of food through your intestinal tract, and by avoiding gas-causing foods such as beans, cabbage, corn, onions and parsnips, fried and other foods that are difficult to digest, and rich desserts. If you use puréed vegetables—the kind which canners prepare for babies—you may obtain some relief. It is also important to chew your food thoroughly to lessen the burden of digesting it.

Hemorrhoids (piles). This is a condition of the blood vessels around the rectum. During pregnancy, the growing uterus may cause pressure in the pelvis and restrict the flow of blood to the area of the rectum. If constipation now occurs, the veins grow larger and more painful under the strain to produce a stool. Sometimes there is slight bleeding.

If you can prevent constipation, you can usually prevent hemorrhoids.

If hemorrhoids become painful, consult your doctor. He may give this advice: Soak a clean cloth in cold witch hazel, ice water or a cold solution of epsom salts. Now lie on your side, with your hips raised on a pillow, and apply the cloth to the rectal region. You may also be advised to use rectal suppositories or to apply an anesthetic ointment to soothe the area of discomfort.

Varicose veins. These also result from the tendency of the expanding uterus to hinder the flow of blood from the lower leg to the abdomen. This results in enlargment of the leg veins just beneath the skin. The condition may become rather painful.

Varicose veins bother first-time mothers much less frequently than pregnant women who have had several children. While it does not seem possible to prevent them entirely, you can follow a program to keep discomfort to a minimum if they develop.

First, eliminate any clothing which tends to hamper circulation. Do not wear round garters or roll your stockings above the knee.

Secondly, keep off your feet as much as possible. Frequent short rest periods in bed or elsewhere in a reclining position with your feet slightly higher than your hips will help the blood flow to your abdomen. Also elevate your legs while reading, watching television, etc.

You can also wear attractive special stockings which help keep the veins from swelling. These stockings should be put on while still in bed in the morning, before the legs are placed in a dependent position and the veins fill, and should be worn as long as you remain on your feet.

Varicose veins will generally disappear after the baby is born when the pressure of your blood vessels disappears.

Leg cramps. Some pregnant women notice cramps in the calf muscles during the later months of pregnancy. These usually occur at night after stretching the leg or turning in bed. While quite painful at the time, they are not of great consequence. They occur most often when the patient has had a busy day on her feet and is tired. The best explanation at present is that the calcium-phosphorus ratio in the body is disturbed. Patients drinking large quantities of milk may be more prone to leg cramps, and it may be necessary to limit the milk intake or take aluminum hydroxide gel to improve the calcium-phosphorus ratio. Massage is of value at the time of cramping and best may be applied with a heating pad, hot water bottle or hot towels.

Abdominal cramps. Abdominal cramps may occur from time to time throughout the pregnancy. They result from the fact that the abdominal muscles must stretch as the fetus grows, and various ligaments in the abdomen are also stretched. So these are literally "growing pains." The best treatment seems to be bed rest, lying on the side of the cramp. The cramps generally pass as quickly as they come. If they persist, your doctor may recommend a special support for your abdomen.

Backaches. As your abdomen expands, your posture changes and more tension will be exerted on your back muscles in order to maintain you in an upright position. Thus a certain amount of backache seems inevitable, especially in the last month, when the size and weight of the abdomen reaches its maximum.

This complaint is more painful than serious. It can be avoided, at least in part, by wearing low-heeled shoes which enable you to balance yourself better when standing or walking, and by wearing a well-fitted maternity girdle. It can be treated by the application of heat; by massaging the affected parts with liniment; and by resting as much as you can.

Shortness of breath. In view of the fact that you will be carrying about fifteen pounds more than your normal weight when your baby is about to be born, you naturally will be unable to engage in some physical activities at that time without feeling shortness of breath. In addition to the extra weight, the uterus may press up against your lungs, making it more difficult to draw a full breath.

Mothers who sometimes have been short of breath in the

seventh month often are agreeably surprised when it disappears two weeks or so before the baby is expected. The explanation is that the infant's head often moves into the pelvis about two weeks before birth, thus relieving pressure against the lungs.

If shortness of breath disturbs your sleep, you may obtain relief by propping up your head with several pillows. If you become short-winded when engaging in activities which are not of a strenuous nature—such as walking a single flight of stairs—mention the fact to your doctor.

Swelling of legs and ankles. Some of your weight increase during pregnancy will result from extra amounts of water retained in the tissues. The water retained, if excessive, goes to the feet and legs, causing them to swell. The best way of dealing with the problem is to elevate your feet at various times throughout the day. The swelling generally recedes after a prolonged rest. Swelling that persists should be reported to your doctor.

Insomnia. Like the inability to sleep that occasionally affects almost everyone, insomnia in pregnancy can result from a wide variety of factors. The basic treatment lies in discovering the specific cause, if possible, and then in removing it.

Many mothers cannot seem to get enough sleep early in pregnancy. When they are bothered by insomnia, it is likely to be in the later stages. A common complaint is that the baby's movements keep the mother awake. The conditions discussed above—heartburn, flatulence, cramps, etc.—may also be contributing factors. Some mothers become obsessed with the thought that they will harm the baby if they sleep in a certain position. Of course, there is no basis in fact for this belief.

If you are unable to sleep, try to isolate the cause—foods which may cause this condition, too much coffee or tea, emotional factors, lack of enough fresh air. Many expectant mothers obtain excellent results by taking a short walk outdoors before retiring. Upon their return, they take a bath or shower, using warm (but not hot) water. Drinking a cup of warm milk just before retiring also helps to induce slumber.

If you cannot seem to isolate the possible causes and are still disturbed by lack of sleep, ask your physician for his recommendation. If conditions warrant, he may prescribe mild sleeping pills to enable you to get the rest you need to carry you through the last few weeks.

Discharge from the vagina. Your doctor may use the term "leucorrhea" to describe this condition. It is normal and to be expected.

During the latter months of pregnancy, the vagina prepares for the role it will play when the baby descends through the birth canal. Instead of secreting the small amount of sticky mucous it normally does—an amount so small you ordinarily do not notice it—the cervical glands now secrete a much larger amount. Along with this secretion, the vagina softens and prepares for the stretching process that will permit the baby to pass through at birth.

If too much mucous is secreted, there may be a vaginal infection. If you wash this area with mild soap and warm water, using a soft cloth, you probably will not be seriously inconvenienced. However, any abnormal increase in the discharge, itching or burning or a changing of its color to yellow or green probably indicates the beginning of an infection. Tell your doctor about it so that he can treat it in its early stages. Never undertake a douche without his specific approval.

Craving for strange foods. One of the legends of pregnancy is that the expectant mother at some unpredictable time can be expected to develop a craving for strange foods she ordinarily would not eat, or for weird combinations like ice cream with pickles. Some doctors say that such strange cravings may merely indicate that the woman feels that she is being neglected and wants more attention than she has been getting. On the other hand, a desire for some foods may indicate that you need the nutritional elements they provide.

Probably no harm is done if you indulge your wishes for certain foods within reason. Your doctor would probably advise against foods which provide little nutritional value and replace those with vitamins and minerals essential for your well-being. Foods high in caloric value should also be taken in moderation. A piece of fruit, which is low in calories, may not give you the same pleasure as the food you fancy but may satisfy your appetite.

COMPLICATIONS OF PREGNANCY

Minor problems in pregnancy may cause discomfort for a time, but probably will cause no permanent harm to yourself or your unborn child. However, there are a few complications of a more serious nature. According to the law of averages, these are unlikely to happen to you. Nevertheless they require prompt attention. Some of these conditions are described below.

German measles. This disease, which goes by the medical name of rubella, appears as a mild and harmless rash. It lasts but a few days. Under ordinary circumstances, it is less troublesome than regular measles, mumps, chicken pox or any of the common diseases of childhood. Only when it strikes in the first three months of pregnancy does it cause special concern.

The significance of German measles in pregnancy was recognized in an Australian study in the early 1940's. In reviewing the histories of mothers who gave birth to babies with physical or mental defects, it was found that many had had German measles early in their pregnancy. From this, it was concluded that the disease produced congenital defects in an alarming percentage of babies born of mothers who had rubella during pregnancy.

Subsequent and recent studies have shown the fallacy of the early Australian work. It is now known that only a small percentage of babies will have major defects if the mother had German measles in the first twelve weeks of the pregnancy. Certain reassuring facts have also been established. For example:

If you had German measles before pregnancy, there is no chance that you will contract it again. As in the case of the more common form of measles, you have developed a lifetime immunity.

If you do not develop German measles during the first twelve weeks of pregnancy, you need not concern yourself about its possible effects on your child. Expectant mothers who have had the disease after that time have no greater percentage of abnormal babies than do other mothers.

If you have not had German measles, therefore, the only period to be concerned about is the first three months of pregnancy. During this period, the wisest course is to avoid associating with anyone who has the disease or has been exposed to it. If you have been exposed to it, you should receive an injection of gamma globulin to prevent you from developing the disease.

It is well to remember that the child of a mother who has had German measles early in her pregnancy has only a slight chance of being affected. Furthermore, most of the effects are of a minor variety. Some busy obstetricians who have managed thousands of pregnancies in their careers can count the number of cases of German measles they have encountered on one hand. And in most cases, the mothers had normal babies.

The Rh factor. Not many years ago, much public interest was focused on this condition. Misunderstanding exists about this subject, too, and it often causes needless concern to mothers—particularly those giving birth for the first time. Briefly, the facts are these:

The Rh factor is a substance in the blood, attached to the red blood cells of about 85 per cent of white people. These people are said to be Rh-positive. Those lacking this substance are Rh-negative. Only about 7 per cent of Negroes are Rh-negative, and about 1 per cent of the yellow race are Rh-negative.

Only mothers with Rh-negative blood may be affected. And trouble arises only when some Rh-positive blood has been introduced into an Rh-negative individual. The mother's blood may then develop antibodies to react to the positive blood. If she conceives a baby with Rh-positive blood, her antibodies may affect the infant's blood and may produce anemia in the infant, through the destruction of red blood cells.

A mother might obtain this incompatible blood by means of a transfusion in the past with Rh-positive blood. But doctors have been aware of this Rh factor for a generation now, and it is unlikely that Rh-positive blood would have been given to any Rh-negative female since about 1942.

The other way a mother might develop these antibodies is by a previous pregnancy, from an infant whose Rh-positive blood she absorbed into her own blood stream. The antibodies created in her system would not be likely to affect her first child but might endanger subsequent ones.

In view of these facts, there is little likelihood that the first child will be troubled by this condition, even if the mother is Rh-negative and the father is Rh-positive.

If your doctor's tests show that you are Rh-positive, you cannot have an "Rh baby." If the test shows your blood to be Rh-negative, however, the doctor will want to determine your husband's Rh status. If your husband's blood is Rh-negative, and you have never had a transfusion of Rh-positive blood, you have no problem at all.

Only if your blood is Rh-negative, and your husband's is Rh-positive, or you have had a transfusion of Rh-positive blood, is there a possibility that you may have an "Rh baby." In that case, your doctor will be prepared to insure your child's safety. He will examine your blood regularly to see if there is any antibody formation. If there is, he may want to deliver the baby a few weeks before the normal time because it is in the latter weeks of pregnancy that the condition becomes most severe. A team of doctors and nurses will be prepared to give an immediate exchange transfusion at the time of delivery to remove the sensitized blood from the infant's system. Following this, such a child should be just as normal as any other infant.

Diabetes in pregnancy. If you suffer from diabetes, the outlook for you and your baby also is good, thanks to modern medical knowledge. However, you will require special treatment. You will need to watch your diet carefully, and be under the careful supervision of a specialist in diabetes.

Your doctor will probably prescribe medications. Working with a specialist in diabetes, he may set down a food list which he will expect you to follow very carefully. This diet will be designed to enable you to meet your basic nutritional requirements, to aid your digestion, and to help you avoid morning sickness, which could be dangerous for a diabetic. He also will test your urine and blood frequently, so as to make sure that the proper sugar balance is maintained and to prevent insulin shock. If you have any trouble in eating, digesting or retaining your food, you should notify the doctor immediately.

Diabetic expectant mothers are now treated so successfully, compared to former years, that almost all of their babies are born in good condition. Some time before the expected date of the arrival, the doctor will decide whether the infant can be delivered vaginally or whether a Caesarean section would be advisable.

The infant will be watched carefully for two or three days after birth and given immediate treatment, if necessary, to insure survival. His outlook should be as good as that of any other child.

Toxemia of pregnancy. This is another condition you need not worry about if you carefully follow your doctor's instructions. If it is untreated, however, it can have very serious consequences for yourself and your unborn child.

The exact nature of toxemia is not fully understood. In fact, it has been called a disease of theories. We recognize it and know how to treat it, but do not know its exact cause. It is characterized by elevated blood pressure, albumin in the urine and swelling of the feet and legs, hands and face.

This condition usually shows up in the last three months of pregnancy. Its symptoms are varied, but the initial sign is usually a rapid increase in weight, with or without obvious swelling. A gain of more than one pound per week should alert you and your doctor before the swelling becomes obvious, and before other symptoms such as headaches, dizziness, blurred vision or vomiting have a chance to develop.

If you have one or more of these symptoms, however, it does not necessarily mean that you have toxemia. But it would be well to report such conditions to your doctor. He will check your blood pressure to see if it has increased since your last visit. He will look for the presence of albumin in the urine—and will check your legs for swelling.

If your physician finds that you have this condition, he will take immediate action. He may hospitalize you, or if the condition is not severe, he may be able to treat you at home. The treatment depends on the severity of the disease. Bed rest, sedatives and diuretics to draw fluid out of your body, a salt-free diet and increased fluid intake, are the principal methods of treatment. If there is no response to therapy, it may be necessary to induce labor or perform a Caesarean section, for the only cure for the disease is to deliver the baby.

Toxemia is usually a passing disturbance without lasting effects, when treated. Once it was a condition which pregnant women bore with various degrees of heroism, and it helped to give pregnancy the reputation of being a difficult time. Today we hear little about its dangers because most women have learned to discuss their symptoms frankly with their doctor— and in sufficient time to enable him to treat the condition.

Pyelitis. This is a urinary-tract infection with which about 2 per cent of expectant mothers are afflicted. It generally develops in the last three months of pregnancy, but may occur at any time during pregnancy.

The simplest explanation is that as the fetus grows, the uterus which contains it enlarges. As the uterus expands, it presses against the ureters through which urine flows from the kidneys to the bladder. If the urine is unable to flow freely the resultant blockade may contribute to infection in the kidneys. Symptoms of pyelitis are chills, fever and pain in either flank which may extend to the lower abdomen.

Your doctor will try to prevent pyelitis by recommending that you drink extra amounts of water all through your pregnancy to help flush the kidneys and to provide a greater volume of urine flow. If you follow his suggestions, you probably will avoid any difficulty of this kind. Should you notice the symptoms of pyelitis, however, notify him at once.

Tuberculosis, heart disease, high blood pressure. A pregnant woman with any of these conditions will naturally require special treatment. But she is in less danger today than at any time before.

Since chest X-rays are no longer routinely done during pregnancy, if there is reason to suspect any chest pathology, your doctor will X-ray your chest. If there is evidence of tuberculosis, a chest specialist will prescribe antibiotics which are highly effective. If surgery is necessary, he will recommend that it be performed during the middle three months of pregnancy.

Women with heart disease today usually come through pregnancy without damage. It is necessary, of course, to adhere strictly to rules laid down by both the obstetrician and the heart specialist. Especially important are rest and diet, and the faithful taking of all prescribed medication.

Your doctor will examine your blood pressure on your first visit and each time thereafter. If it is high, it can be kept within safe limits with drugs developed within the past few years. The doctor will recommend a special diet designed to limit both your calories and your salt intake.

Threatened miscarriage. Laymen use the term "miscarriage" to describe the expulsion of a fetus from the mother's womb usually before the third month of pregnancy. Your doctor may use the word "abortion" for the same thing, but this term does not mean that any moral guilt is involved. The word "abortion," when used in this sense, is usually preceded by the word "spontaneous," meaning that it occurred without the mother's desire or help. If she took deliberate steps to cause the miscarriage, it would be properly described as "criminal" abortion—a violation of the law of God and of the State as well.

Do not be alarmed over the danger of miscarriage. It has been estimated that 10 per cent of all pregnancies end in this way, but they generally occur before the third month and the mother usually feels no great physical pain. Considerably fewer miscarriages occur after the third month.

A miscarriage generally is a tragedy because it runs counter to a woman's normal desire for motherhood. Nevertheless, there should be consolation in the thought that when miscarriage occurs early in the pregnancy, almost always there is some condition which might cause a child to be defective in some way. Thus, loss of the embryo may be more of a blessing than a young mother realizes, for nature has acted so that she will not be burdened with a child who might be lacking in some essentials.

When a mother miscarries early in pregnancy, most medical authorities hold, there is little she could have done to prevent it. Thus she can accept the event as the expression of a Higher Will over which she has had no control.

What occurs in miscarriage is that the placenta separates from the uterus. This separation may be slight, in which case bed rest may help the placenta to retain its hold. After it has reached a certain point, however, the loosening will continue until the entire placenta is free of the uterus. At that point it may be totally or partially discharged. Since it takes up to about fourteen weeks for the placenta and membranes to be firmly attached, it is during the early stages that miscarriage is most likely to occur.

Once a fetus develops beyond the fifth or sixth month, a mother can do much to make sure that she will carry the baby to full term. Experience has shown that some miscarriages in the later stages result from falls, excessive work and fatigue, lifting of heavy objects, and accidents. So simple common sense demands that you take all reasonable precautions, avoid heavy work or long automobile rides, and get adequate rest.

One woman actually laid concrete blocks to help build her own home well into the last month of her pregnancy. She did manual labor, beyond the powers of many men, without ill effects. On the other hand, another woman—seemingly just as strong physically—slipped off a low bathroom stool and had a miscarriage. Unfortunately, we cannot exactly tell in advance who is susceptible to miscarriage, nor who could work from dawn to dusk in the fields—as pioneer women did—without trouble.

The reasonable procedure, therefore, is to follow your doctor's recommendations. He will probably advise you to keep off your feet as much as possible, avoid excessive physical activity, and try to develop a calm and serene attitude. He may use other means to minimize the danger of miscarriage if he thinks that they are needed. He may prescribe hormones which your body needs for full growth of the fetus.

You should learn to recognize the danger signs indicating that miscarriage may be beginning. The first and most important of these is bleeding, or staining, from the vagina. If you observe even the slightest sign of it, you should lie down immediately and be sure to telephone your doctor. He may prescribe drugs which help hold back the miscarriage process if it has just started. By staying in bed, you may be able to pass through the period successfully and get up after a few days and go about your business.

Continued bleeding may indicate that the fetus and placenta are being discharged. Usually there will be crampy pain in the lower abdomen. If the fetus and placenta are not passed in their entirety, a minor operation at the hospital may be necessary. It is a curettage—a scraping out of any tissue which remains in the uterus after the expulsion of the fetus. The curettage is perofrmed under anesthesia and is therefore painless.

In spontaneous miscarriage of this type, tissue or clots from the vagina should be kept for the doctor to examine. From these, he may be able to tell much about the cause, and perhaps help the patient to prevent a similar occurrence the next time.

In most cases, the embryo or fetus has died in the uterus as a result of the separation of the placenta from the uterine wall, and may or may not be recognized as such, when passed out of the body.

In some cases, however, the fetus may be alive and may live for a short time. When this occurs, the Catholic mother should see to it that the fetus is baptized. The Church teaches that anyone—regardless of his or her own religious beliefs—may perform the Sacrament of Baptism. He or she merely pours water over the head of the infant while pronouncing the words, "If you are alive, I baptize thee in the name of the Father, and of the Son and of the Holy Ghost."

A woman who has had a spontaneous abortion in the first three months of pregnancy generally can embark on another pregnancy after two or three normal menstrual cycles. Since the miscarriage was probably the result of a poor sperm or poor egg and probably not a defect in her body, the situation next time might be entirely different.

If miscarriage occurs later in the pregnancy, however, the doctor may conclude that conditions inside the mother's body were responsible. He may suggest that these conditions be remedied before another attempt is made to conceive.

If a woman has three miscarriages, and all at about the same period in her pregnancy, a condition of habitual abortion is said to exist. Under these circumstances, her doctor will try to trace physical or emotional reasons which may be responsible. He may put his patient on a high-protein, high-vitamin diet, rich in vitamin C, and will probably investigate thyroid function and take special X-rays of the uterus.

Since psychological factors are sometimes believed to lie behind repeated miscarriages, a patient with this history should not feel that her doctor is prying into her personal affairs if he questions her about her psychological problems, her relations with her husband, and so on. That is why you should always feel free to tell your innermost fears to your doctor, knowing that he will view your problems sympathetically and in the strictest confidence. Sometimes a patient's hidden concerns may keep her from successful pregnancy. Her adviser may be able to convince her that her worries have no genuine basis in fact.

A doctor will generally suggest a very conservative routine for a patient with repeated miscarriages. He may wish her to give up habits or avoid situations or people which cause her a great deal of emotional tension. He may advise her to get extra bed rest during periods when she is especially vulnerable to miscarriage. He may urge her to avoid intercourse all through the pregnancy or at times when she has been prone to miscarriage in the past. He may propose other restrictions—avoidance of drinking or smoking or elimination of certain physical activities like gardening. The woman who visits him before she becomes pregnant, follows his instructions faithfully, and tries to cultivate a serene, hopeful outlook, will greatly enhance her chances of carrying her baby to full term. Many women have several miscarriages, then go on to bear a large number of children.

Deliberate abortions. It may be assumed that as a reader of this book, you wish to do all within your power to give birth to a happy, normal child. Thus the thought of induced abortion is alien to this discussion—especially deliberate abortion in which a child is destroyed to suit the convenience of the mother.

Such abortion is murder, of course; it violates both the law of God and of the country. No reputable doctor would perform such an operation. Whether performed by midwives, or by doctors who have already lost their license to practice or would lose it if they were discovered, these operations are dangerous. They are generally done in unsanitary surroundings and without benefit of the life-saving equipment which a modern hospital provides. They may cause permanent physical damage to the woman. They may also leave deep psychological scars, for she may well develop a deep sense of shame when she realizes that she has been a party to an act that has denied her very nature—an act contrary to her deepest God-given instincts.

In some hospitals, however, doctors perform "therapeutic abortions"—in which the fetus is forcibly removed from the uterus because of fears that the mother's health might be endangered if the pregnancy proceeded naturally. It is our view, of course, that human life exists from the moment the male sperm unites with the female ovum. Therefore, destroying that tiny life is as wrong as any deliberate attempt upon the life of an adult human being anywhere.

From the medical viewpoint alone, there is very little justification for "therapeutic" abortions. In fact, few obstetricians have ever encountered a case in which they could state with absolute certainty that a mother would die if she carried a child until it could be born alive. True, there are some conditions—severe heart disease, hypertension, nephritis, etc.—where it may be more dangerous for a woman to have a child than it would be normally. But the mortality rate from childbirth, even for women with the most serious conditions, is almost negligible today. Even a woman in extremely poor physical condition has an excellent chance of survival.

In some hospitals, there are physicians who admittedly perform an abortion when it is not a question of the mother's life, but only of her health. For example, some doctors abort a woman when she is mentally disturbed and they believe her condition might worsen if she has a baby. Some suggest abortion if the mother suffers from cancer of the breast or cervix, or from diabetes or the toxemias of pregnancy. But few obstetricians would state categorically that the mother would die if she carried her baby to viability.

It is true that in such instances, the mother's life would be in less jeopardy if she were not pregnant. But pregnancy involves some risk for any woman—even a healthy, normal one.

It is also well to remember that when a woman suffers from

a disease so serious that her life may be threatened, such as cancer, a doctor may morally use every therapeutic means at his command to save her life—even if the fetus should die as an *indirect* result of the treatment. As a practical matter, therefore, the question of "mother or child" does not arise.

Many cases might be cited of women who were told that they should have a "therapeutic abortion" because giving birth would jeopardize their health. They consulted other doctors who assured them that they could carry their babies to full term without undue risk. Now their children are a source of satisfaction and comfort. Had they succumbed to abortion, they would not now know the joys of parenthood, and they would be haunted by the memory of what they had done. One Catholic hospital in New York takes many of the most difficult obstetrical cases to be found, including patients who have left other doctors who suggested abortions. Of some 6,000 cases, it has had but one fatality, proving that good medicine and good morals are not contradictory.

Most obstetricians will respect your religious convictions in this matter. If you are asked to go against your moral beliefs, ask your moral adviser to guide you. Also remember that you are always free, at any time during your pregnancy, to consult another doctor.

The evil of sterilization. Some cases which are falsely thought to justify abortion are also used to justify sterilization of the woman. It is argued that it will always be unsafe for her to bear children, and therefore sterilization—a second violation of the moral laws—is performed at the same time as the abortion.

The damage of sterilization can rarely be undone. The usual method of sterilization is to tie the Fallopian tubes to prevent future movement of the female egg into the uterus. It can no longer unite with the male sperm and conception thereafter is impossible.

The woman who submits to this operation destroys a part of herself. She may never bear a child again—no matter how much her health may improve, or how desperately she may desire to fulfill her normal functions of motherhood. The emotional harm can hardly be overestimated. The deep sense of loss a woman may feel when she realizes that she has permitted a basic part of her nature to be taken away far outweighs any physical benefits that might result.

When to call your doctor immediately. As the above review indicates, most pregnancies are free of complications which might affect your well-being or that of your child. However, certain indications should be reported to your doctor at once. If you learn to recognize the signals and call them to his attention immediately, he can treat them in the early stages and avoid possible difficulties later.

Call him at once if you observe one or more of the following conditions:

1. Any severe vomiting or nausea, or vomiting or nausea that continues for any length of time.

2. A headache that does not respond to common, ordinary treatment, or that is either more severe or more prolonged than usual, or that manifests itself in ways you have not experienced before.

3. Any swelling or puffed-up feeling around your face, eyes or hands.

4. Any pronounced swelling of your feet or ankles that does not go down after a night's rest, or that shows itself soon after you get on your feet in the morning.

5. Any blurring of your vision, dimness, or the appearance of spots before your eyes.

6. Pronounced increase or decrease in the amount of urine you pass.

7. Any pain or burning sensation while passing urine.

8. Any chills or fever. Normal body temperature is 98.6 degrees on a thermometer placed in the mouth. Any temperature exceeding 99.6, when accompanied by other symptoms, however slight, should be reported.

9. Sharp or continuous pains in your abdomen.

10. Bleeding from the vagina, no matter how slight. However, do not mistake for this an increase in the discharge of vaginal mucous which is normal in pregnancy.

11. Any gush of water from the vagina. This may indicate the bursting of the membranes surrounding the baby and may indicate that labor is about to begin.

Your obstetrician can be reached at any hour of the day or night. If you call when he is not in his office the message will be taken by someone who will get in touch with him as soon as possible.

When phoning your doctor, have a pencil and paper at hand so that you can write down any instructions he may give. Also have ready for instant reference the name, address and telephone number of your pharmacist. The doctor may want to phone a prescription to the pharmacist so that it can be prepared and delivered to your home without unnecessary delay.

While waiting to speak to your physician, you should not be excessively disturbed by your symptoms. Even if several occur simultaneously, they may not indicate serious danger. Let your doctor be the judge of that. But by calling his attention to these "danger signals" when they appear, you are insuring that if special treatment is needed, he will give it and there will be less danger of more severe complications. If at all possible, speak to the doctor yourself, because only you can answer his questions properly. Besides the time saved, something may be misinterpreted when the questions and answers go through a third party. It is a rare occasion when you are unable to speak directly to your doctor.

DECISIONS YOU MUST MAKE BEFORE THE BABY COMES

Is natural childbirth for you? You may wish to consider having your baby by the method popularized by Dr. Grantly Dick Read of England. His phrase "Natural Childbirth" has gained acceptance into the language but many obstetricians in England, the United States and elsewhere feel that it does not adequately express the method which he espouses. A chief principle of natural childbirth is that many of a pregnant woman's fears—and the pain she experiences in labor—can be averted if she has been thoroughly prepared, psychologically and physically, for the process of giving birth.

Natural childbirth involves first of all what you are doing now—gaining an increased knowledge of pregnancy, an understanding of what actually happens when you conceive, as the fetus develops, and finally when you actually give birth. If you know about these things and feel free to discuss with your doctor any questions which arise, you undoubtedly will have greater peace of mind. Your knowledge will give you a sense of security and will reduce, if not eliminate, the tension you might feel about your condition. If you can adopt a more relaxed attitude toward your pregnancy—an attitude which generally comes from knowledge—you will also increase your ability to endure the physical strain of childbirth.

One aspect of natural childbirth consists in preparing the body for labor and delivery. Primarily, this is done by exercises which develop the muscles used in giving birth. Expectant mothers also are taught breathing exercises to enable them to endure better the contractions of the uterus which occur during labor and continue until the baby is delivered. In natural childbirth, a well-prepared mother may remain awake during the delivery if she desires. She feels an intimate joy of participation in this great moment when her baby draws his first breath. However, any patient who needs relief from pain can obtain such drugs during labor and may have anesthesia for the actual delivery.

Some years ago, Pope Pius XII dispelled any doubts about the Church's position on natural childbirth. He declared that "the instruction given in regard to nature's travail in childbirth; the correction of false interpretations of organic sensations and the invitation to correct them; the influence exercised to avoid groundless anxiety and fear; the assistance afforded the mother in childbirth opportunely to collaborate with nature, to remain tranquil and under self-control; an increased consciousness of the greatness of motherhood in general, and particularly of the hour when the mother brings forth her child—all these are positive values to which no reproach can be made. They are benefits for the mother in childbirth and fully conform to the will of the Creator."

If you are interested you might ask your doctor about it early in your pregnancy, probably in the first half. His own experiences with mothers in natural childbirth may be the best guide for you. A question of personality also is involved. What may be best for one woman may be unsuited for another. Whether you could obtain the necessary training in your community must also be considered.

Values of breast-feeding. Sometime before your baby is expected, you should also decide whether you will attempt to feed him from your breasts. A generation ago, breast-feeding was somewhat unpopular. Preparing formulas and feeding babies from the bottle seemed the smart thing to do. In recent years, however, there has been a decided swing back to breast-feeding. There are many reasons for this trend.

Most important is the fact that it is the natural way to feed a baby. His mother's milk contains the nutritional values he needs and also has a substance that helps his digestive processes. If the mother herself has a proper diet, it has a good composition of the necessary vitamins, minerals, and proteins.

Breast-feeding has a great psychological value for the baby. It is important to realize that the process of being born involves one of the greatest shocks a human being experiences. In the womb, the fetus is fed, kept secure from extremes of heat and cold, and is always sheltered. When the baby is born, he enters a strange world where he must immediately learn to breathe for himself, to eat, to endure some heat or some cold, and so on. Psychologists tell us that in these initial stages, the sense of security he felt in the womb can best be given to him if he is often held close to the mother, enclosed in the warmth and protection of her arms.

Breast-feeding also helps the mother physically and psychologically. It helps restore her childbearing organs to their normal state, and gives her the feeling that she is giving something of herself to help her baby's growth. This feeling intensifies the joys of motherhood, and makes her realize that any sacrifice she must make to help her child grow to adulthood will be worth while. Many mothers have said that one of the greatest satisfactions they have known is the feeling of trust and love they see in the eyes of the infant at the breast.

Three common objections to breast-feeding. Young women sometimes object to breast-feeding on three grounds: that it may be embarrassing, may cause them to lose their figures, and may tie them down unnecessarily.

Of course, breast-feeding cannot be indecent because it was

the means which God ordained to provide nourishment for the newly born. Nor need women who wear special maternity brassieres ordinarily fear that they will lose their figures. Nor does breast-feeding tie down the mother who plans to care for her baby herself. In fact, one survey of young mothers showed that those who breast-fed considered themselves less tied down than did those who had to carry an array of sterilizers, materials for formulas, baby bottles and similar items wherever they went. Of course, breast-feeding is not practical for the mother who intends to work soon after the baby is born or who has many interests outside the home.

Take your doctor's advice. There may be medical reasons applicable in your case why he will advise you against breast-feeding. A general opinion now, however, is that mothers should try it if they are so inclined. However, if you do not wish to breast-feed, or find that your supply of milk is insufficient, do not be upset and do not consider yourself a failure. Rest assured that with today's formulas your baby can thrive just as well as a breast-fed baby. As far as the psychological effect on the baby is concerned, there are many outstanding physicians who feel that it is not the source of the milk which makes a difference, but the manner in which the baby is fed. A baby held close to its mother, enclosed in the warmth and protection of her arms, and given a bottle instead of the breast, receives the same love and careful attention which it needs for its sense of security. A bottle propped on a pillow, however, is a poor substitute for a mother's arms.

To breast-feed successfully, you and your baby must spend a few days adjusting to it, but a normal infant generally draws sufficient milk from the breasts within a few days. Some mothers cannot provide all the milk their babies need and additional formula feedings are necessary. It has been found that the best nursers are confident, placid mothers with a good emotional adjustment and an earnest desire to feed the baby, and who do not become tired or upset easily.

Should you work after your baby is born? Not many years ago, this question probably would not have been asked. If asked, it would have been answered with a resounding "no." A mother's place was thought to be by her baby's side, not in paid employment outside the home.

As a result of the emancipation of women, however, the question now is not only asked, but even answered by some experts in the affirmative. A little consideration of your baby's needs should convince you, however, that you will serve him best by taking care of him yourself.

First of all, only you can give the continuity of care and affection that he needs. For his proper emotional development, your baby must have the sense of security that comes from developing a trust in one person who will constantly attend to his needs. A mother who works outside the home cannot give this attention. Even if she obtains a devoted nurse as a substitute, there is always the possibility that the nurse will change employment and that the baby will be cared for by a succession of different persons.

Generally speaking, only a mother can give the constant affection and tender guidance a child needs for his good emotional development. A study on this subject was made under the direction of Dr. John Bowlby, a famed British expert. Dr. Bowlby reported that when a baby learns to give his love to one person, who consistently takes care of him, he develops that trust in human beings which he must have in order to deal confidently with other people throughout his life.

The importance of having a mother to love—rather than a mother-substitute—was poignantly but dramatically illustrated in England during World War II. Some London children were sent by their parents to rural areas where they would be safe from enemy bombings. Others remained in the midst of the target areas, but with their mothers. Those in charge of the program naturally regarded the evacuated youngsters as the favored ones. But when they compared records of the two groups, they learned that children who remained with their mothers had fewer cases of mental and emotional disturbance than did those presumably beyond harm's reach. The conclusion was inescapable: A mother's love gives a child more security than anything else that can be given him.

This is the fundamental point you might consider if you believe that by working outside the home you can give your child a few luxuries he might otherwise have to do without. For your attention and love are as necessary to him as food and shelter. They should not be given up for the sake of things which are unnecessary for his development as a well-adjusted person.

Wise mothers who could easily afford to have their children cared for by others recognize the importance of this personal attention. They realize that no satisfaction in life will equal that which comes from playing an intimate part in every step of a baby's growth. It was this realization that was behind Mrs. John F. Kennedy's statement at the time of her husband's election to the Presidency that it was a drawback of his election that her official duties might cut down the amount of time she could give to the personal care of her children. Many other mothers in somewhat similar positions realize that their highest duty is to give of themselves personally in the upbringing of their own families.

If you have no choice but to return to work after your baby is born, and this would be the exceptional case, try to get someone to care for him who can hold the position for many years if necessary. Your own blood relatives may be a better choice than hired nurses who might discontinue their employment at any time. Avoid a constant succession of caretakers, all with ways strange to him. He will have no one to whom he can give a confident continuity of trust.

Arranging for your hospital stay. Several months before the expected date of delivery, you should select the hospital for your confinement. You will be asked to choose one at which your doctor ordinarily practices. Some hospitals have a small selected group of doctors to whom they make their facilities available, and here there is usually no problem about reservations. At other hospitals, however, where a large number of doctors have privileges, you must make reservations several months in advance in order to be sure of a room when your time comes for delivery.

A generation or two ago, expectant mothers often felt that they had a choice between a hospital delivery and one at home. Since then, hospital deliveries have become the usual thing. Unless you live several hours away from a hospital—an unlikely circumstance in these days of fast cars and good roads —you should have your baby where modern equipment will insure your safety and that of your baby, and where a staff of doctors and nurses will see that you get the best care available.

Clothes and accessories you will need. You will not require many articles of clothing or personal items in the hospital. Here are probably all you will need: bathrobe, bedroom slippers, several nightgowns, bed jacket, nursing brassieres, sanitary belt, and such toilet articles as comb, brush, hand mirror, cosmetics, face powder, toothbrush, toothpaste and facial tissues.

You may want to pack a fountain pen, pencils, stationery, address book and stamps. Some expectant mothers buy a supply of birth announcements before the baby is born, and address and stamp the envelopes at their leisure. After the baby arrives, they merely fill in details and send the announcements on their way before they leave the hospital.

You might also bring along some reading matter—perhaps

a book or two dealing with the care of your child. One on the spiritual aspects of parenthood might make inspiring reading during your convalescence.

The hospital probably will provide gowns for you to wear before and for a few days after the baby is born. It will also provide the diapers and other garments your baby will need in the hospital. For this reason, you need not worry if you must hurry off to the hospital without having everything packed. Your husband will have ample time to bring the things you will need for yourself and the baby.

Several weeks before the estimated date of delivery, you might pack the clothes the baby will wear when he leaves the hospital. Put the package aside so that your husband will be able to take it to you a day or so before you are scheduled to return home. This bundle might contain several diapers, one undershirt, several large safety pins, a petticoat and dress or other outer wrapper, a sweater, cap and blankets. The amount of clothes the baby will need to keep warm will depend upon the weather. On a wintry day, he may need both a sweater and either a heavy bunting or warm blanket.

You might also carefully set aside your own clothes which you will want to wear home from the hospital because otherwise it might take two or three expeditions before the correct clothes can finally be found and brought to the hospital.

WHAT KIND OF BABY WILL YOU HAVE?

Will your baby have his father's hair or his mother's eyes? Will he inherit his uncle's musical talents? What are your chances of having twins? Can we tell if the baby will be a boy or girl?

Prospective mothers and fathers frequently ask many questions like these about the baby they are likely to have. Here are answers to the most common ones.

Will your baby be normal? The mathematical odds are overwhelming that he will be. Most likely, his mind and intellect will be in the middle group of people who are neither mentally retarded at one extreme nor exceptionally gifted at the other. He will probably be physically normal as well. But the odds are also heavily against your having a "perfect baby." Like their parents, most children have minor defects. One may not have a fully symmetrical figure or face. Another may inherit a tendency toward skin trouble. A third may be color-blind, or suffer from allergies.

The point is that you will be disappointed if you fail to allow for the fact that your baby will probably be less than perfect. There will be areas—physical, mental or emotional—in which you can strengthen him. You will be better able to accept him as he is if you recognize the fact in advance that in being normal, he will not be perfect. About one child in every hundred is exceptionally gifted and has mental equipment far superior to the average. Perhaps one in several hundred might be called a "genius."

Usually, a child's mental superiority does not manifest itself until he is a year old, and you may not have real proof of it until he is nine or ten. The superior child generally learns to take care of himself, and to talk, read and count at an earlier age than the average. He tends to be a questioner—one who continually asks "why?" He often picks up unusual words and enjoys using them in conversation. He may have an exceptional memory.

Some parents mistakenly think that a bright child is difficult to raise. However, the belief that a "child prodigy" is likely to grow up as a useless citizen is not founded in fact. Careful studies have shown that gifted children generally adjust better to life, have happier marriages and develop fewer vices than do children of normal intelligence.

The best way to encourage your child's intellectual development—whether he is "normal" or "superior"—is to encourage him to read extensively in subjects in which he is interested, to develop his intellectual bents such as building or collecting things, and to do those things for which he shows strong aptitudes.

What are the chances that your baby will be mentally retarded? The odds are roughly one hundred to one in favor of your having a normal youngster. Of course, every parent faces the possibility that the infant may not measure up mentally. Even an infant born to a man and woman who are highly gifted intellectually may be retarded, while the child of parents of below-average intelligence may have a superior intellect.

It is now generally realized that the birth of a retarded baby is no reflection on his parents. They should be prepared to accept any child which God in His Divine Wisdom gives them, and to give love and affection to their infant regardless of his strong or weak points.

Tremendous steps in the past few years have been made in treating handicapped children. Improvements in their condition which are now commonplace would have been considered impossible a dozen or so years ago. Loving parents can enable a youngster to build a successful life despite his handicap. The birth of a retarded child therefore should not be considered as a defeat for the parents but rather as a challenge.

Where do the baby's "inherited characteristics" come from? Difficult as it may be to believe, they are all determined by the microscopic cells which come from the mother and father. Some idea of the size involved might be gleaned from the fact that an ordinary tablespoon would hold about two million female eggs, and that the male sperm is about one five-hundredth of an inch long. It is believed that these germ cells contain about thirty thousand genes, which carry the characteristics passed down from generation to generation. Such characteristics will include the color of skin and eyes, more than average proficiency in mathematics, special talents for music, and the like.

The baby's sex is determined by the male sperm. The amount deposited by the male into the vagina generally consists of about an equal number of female-producing and male-producing sperm. If X-type sperm unites with the egg of the female, a girl will result. If Y-type of sperm fertilizes the egg, a boy will result.

What characteristics of yours will your baby inherit? While the complete answer is not fully known, scientists now believe that your child will inherit the kind of physical characteristics which you have inherited—but not those which you have acquired in your own lifetime. To illustrate:

One infant's parents were blue-eyed redheads. He too was a blue-eyed redhead, and there was no doubt that he inherited the characteristics from his parents. On the other hand, another infant's father suffered from a childhood disease which left him partially deaf. There was no likelihood that his child would inherit this acquired characteristic.

Your children will resemble you in many ways. The chances are that a brilliant professor's son will have a higher native intelligence than the son of an unskilled laborer, and that a boy born of a long line of athletes will be more athletic than one whose parents and grandparents led very passive physical lives. These are inherited characteristics. But there is no certainty that these conditions will exist in all cases.

The example you show your child in his everyday life will have an important effect on his development—but it cannot affect the native talents with which he was born originally.

His environment may enable him to use these talents more or less effectively, but it cannot change their innate existence.

What characteristics "run in families"? You might predict some of your baby's characteristics if you consider the outstanding ones his father and mother have. If both mother and father are short, the children will probably be short—but chances are they will be taller than their parents because we now know more about good nutrition, which aids growth. If both parents have blue eyes, their children will probably be blue-eyed. When both are dark-eyed, most of the children will be dark-eyed. When one parent is blue-eyed, the other dark-eyed, chances are greater that the baby will have blue eyes. The same situation prevails in the case of hair. If a blonde and brunette marry, it is more likely that the baby will be blonde.

In such cases, the trait that shows up more often in a matching of two characteristics is called dominant. The trait which is less likely to appear is known as recessive.

This question of inheritance is extremely complicated. The important point to remember is that neither you nor your husband can do anything about certain characteristics your child will have. If they are favorable characteristics, however, you can use them and take advantage of them. If they are not so desirable, you can develop them so that they are less of a problem or cease to be one at all.

Can diseases of the parents be inherited? With the exception of a few diseases—for example, albinism and a rare type of hemophilia which makes it difficult or impossible to stop bleeding once it begins—most diseases are not inherited. However, some diseases—such as syphilis—may be acquired from an infected mother. If the infection is treated during or before pregnancy, the baby will not contract it.

However, he may inherit a tendency toward a certain disease

—a constitutional weakness or predisposition which may make him more likely to contract it unless proper precautions are taken. Diabetes and tuberculosis are believed to fall in this category.

Which is more important for your baby—his heredity or his environment? This question often starts much controversy. A favorite answer of scientists is that "heredity deals the cards, but environment plays the hand." As in a bridge game, the alert parent can often get better results with a poor child than the inept parent can get with a good one.

You cannot do anything about your child's heredity at this stage but by providing a good environment you can help him achieve the full potential of his natural endowments. As his mother, you will have the greatest power to encourage his use of whatever gifts God has given him.

What are your chances of having twins? Odds are about 90 to 1 that you will not have twins in any given pregnancy; about 7,500 to 1 that you will not have triplets; about 700,000 to 1 that you will not have four babies at once; and 60,000,000 to 1 that you will not have quintuplets.

You are more likely to have twins if there is a history of them in your family—if you were a twin yourself, or your brothers and sisters were twins.

There are three kinds of twins: identical twins—the result of one ovum which has divided in two; nonidentical twins of the same sex, when two ova were fertilized at the same time or almost the same time; and non-identical twins of opposite sexes from two ova which also were fertilized almost simultaneously. Single-ovum twinning occurs most frequently in women between the ages of twenty and thirty-five and occurs with the same frequency that would be expected were it just a chance phenomenon, irrespective of whether it was the first or third or fifth pregnancy.

However, double-ovum twinning is characteristic of older women and those who already have two or more children.

Inasmuch as identical twins are the product of the same ovum which has been fertilized by the one sperm, each child receives an identical inheritance. Such twins will grow up looking much alike. Differences they develop as they grow up will be the result of environmental factors.

Can twins be predicted in advance? In a practical sense, it usually is possible to predict a multiple birth only after the fifth or sixth month, when the doctor can hear the heartbeat with his stethoscope. If he hears two separate heartbeats, he naturally can conclude you will have twins. He may also be able to determine this by feeling your abdomen. If he thinks it necessary, he may have X-rays taken to establish the fact beyond doubt.

Is it possible to determine the baby's sex before birth? At this time scientists know of no accurate way to do this that is simple enough for practical clinical use. It is known, of course, that the baby's sex is determined at the moment of conception, and that this depends upon whether the female egg is fertilized by a male-producing sperm or a female-producing one. But there is no easy way to tell the sex until the baby actually is born.

While "hoping" for a boy or girl is a harmless diversion, some parents build their expectations too high. As a result, they may be severely disappointed if the sex is not the one they hoped for. In extreme cases, some parents express their disappointment by treating the child unfairly, as though the baby somehow were responsible. A more reasonable attitude seems to be that either a boy or girl will be welcome and that you will be grateful for whatever God chooses to give.

Can the baby be "marked" as a result of an accident during pregnancy? This is an old belief, but lacks any scientific foundation. Your emotional reactions during pregnancy cannot affect the appearance of your child. Birthmarks result from influences over which parents have no known control.

If your child has birthmarks, they are likely to be of little or no consequence. If they are large, you might ask your doctor what can be done about them.

THE BIRTH OF YOUR BABY

Significant signs before labor. You may notice a pronounced shift in your baby's position about two weeks before the expected birth date. He will seem to have moved down lower in your abdomen, relieving pressure on your stomach and lungs. If you have experienced heartburn, you may now find that the condition has been suddenly relieved. What has happened is that the baby's head has begun to move into your pelvic canal so that it will be ready for its journey into the world when your actual labor begins.

No one is absolutely sure why labor begins when it does. Many theories have been expressed but no one theory finds all doctors in complete accord. It is known, of course, that abnormal conditions—such as accidents, shock, and high fever—may cause premature labor. Normally, however, there is no such dramatic or specific event to mark the starting point.

During pregnancy, there are regular, periodic contractions of the uterus which may cause no discomfort and have no significant effect. Toward the end of pregnancy, however, these contractions may become stronger and more regular.

Before labor begins, you may feel a slight pain as the uterus contracts. When this occurs, the head of the fetus may be moving deeper into the pelvis and there may be some dilation of the cervix, the lower end of the uterus. Expectant mothers sometimes notice these contractions at night and may mistakenly think that labor is beginning. The commonly known term "false labor" describes this condition.

Another sign that pregnancy is coming to an end is the enlargement of the vulva. The patient begins to sense congestion in that region.

A more imminent sign is "the show." This is a mucous discharge, with streaks of blood. "The show" is generally a fairly reliable indication that actual labor will soon begin—probably within several hours.

Six signs that actual labor is beginning. Learn to recognize the characteristics of labor. When associated with dilatation of the cervix, these are evidence that you will soon give birth. There are six signs to remember:

1. The contractions of the uterus are generally painful.

2. They are involuntary—beyond your control. At first, they are generally felt in the lower back or lower abdomen.

3. They are peristaltic in nature—similar to the cramps that some women feel at menstruation.

4. Each contraction is prolonged. It is generally faint at the beginning, gradually rises to a peak, then fades away.

5. The contractions are rhythmic. At the beginning of labor you may feel them every twenty minutes or so. Gradually the interval between them becomes shorter and shorter.

6. As labor progresses, the contractions will occur more frequently, will be more intense and will last longer.

During intervals between contractions, you may feel completely comfortable. You may feel sleepy and may even be able to doze off. But it is wise to notify your doctor when you believe labor has begun. He will want to know how often the contractions are coming. To do this, you time from the start of one contraction to the start of the next one, and also note how long the contractions last. Do not try to estimate but actually use a watch.

One girl who realized the value of prayer, when asked how often the contractions were coming, replied, "Oh, about every three Hail Marys." Fortunately she prayed slowly and made it to the hospital on time.

After discussing the situation with you, he will tell you whether you should go the hospital immediately or how long you should wait before going.

Along about the eighth month of pregnancy, of course, you should have listed the garments, personal toilet articles, etc., that you plan to take to the hospital with you, and you should now be ready to pack your bag and leave your home upon a few minutes' notice.

Getting to the hospital. You should have made your plans for transportation a month or so before the expected date. Preferably, your husband should accompany you. But you should have arranged with relatives or friends to go with you if labor began in his absence. Or you should have listed in a handy place the phone numbers of taxicab companies or private ambulance services you might call.

While you probably will have ample time to get to the hospital before more severe labor begins, you may not have enough time to dress and make up completely. You will be forgiven on this occasion if you are not as well groomed as usual.

Some patients become unduly excited when labor begins. They fear that they may give birth in a taxicab or under other unusual circumstances. Remember that such deliveries are extremely rare—so much so, in fact, that such a birth generally makes front-page news when it occurs.

Considerably before this time, either you or your doctor will have advised the hospital you have selected that you will be a patient about this time. As soon as he directs you to leave for the hospital, he will also phone the institution and advise them that you will soon make your appearance.

When you suspect that you are entering labor, avoid eating any solid food. If anesthesia is needed to help you in childbirth, it can be dangerous with a full stomach, because of possible vomiting and aspiration of food particles into the lungs.

At the hospital, if you have not already done so, you will be asked to provide basic facts about yourself for the institution's record—your age, religion, whether you have hospitalization insurance, and similar information. Sometimes expectant mothers and fathers are annoyed by what appears to be the brisk, unconcerned attitude of nurses and attendants. Of course, nurses are concerned for your welfare. But they know that childbirth is a normal process, and although it may be exciting and possibly even frightening to you, it is something that they deal with every day and take in stride. They know that there is little likelihood that you will deliver while giving routine information at the admitting desk. To alleviate this situation, some hospitals have a form, given you by your doctor beforehand, which you simply present on admission.

Within a few minutes, you will be taken to the labor room you will occupy. You will be asked to undress, or helped to do so by a nurse, if necessary. Next, you will be prepared and possibly given an enema. By now, your doctor may be at the hospital. He will examine you thoroughly to determine the position of the fetus in the womb and to make certain that the neck of the cervix is dilating so that the baby's head can pass through. He will remain at the hospital, or will be nearby so that he can quickly reach your side to help you as labor progresses.

The three stages of labor. Labor is generally divided into three distinct parts—dilatation of the cervix, explusion of the baby, and expulsion of the placenta. The dilation stage starts when the uterus begins to contract on a regular, rhythmic basis. During this time the cervix dilates and the head descends, so that the fetus will be able to pass along with a minimum of difficulty. The second stage begins when the cervix is fully dilated and ends when the baby has completely emerged from his mother's body. The third stage occurs when the placenta and surrounding membranes are expelled. When this happens, the uterus contracts to prevent bleeding and the birth process is completed.

How long will you be in labor? It is difficult to say in advance because the length of labor varies a great deal. However, some researchers have found that the average woman labors about fifteen hours with her first child, and about ten hours with succeeding ones. These figures may not be reliable indicators in your case, because some women make very rapid progress in labor while others require more time than the average. It is true in a general way, however, that the younger you are when you have your first baby, the shorter the duration of labor.

Is it true that you must have a specified number of labor pains before your baby is born? This is apparently another belief, handed down from generation to generation, which has no specific scientific evidence to back it up. Doctors have noted tremendous differences, depending upon a wide variety of factors, in the number, extent and duration of contractions which mothers have experienced.

It does seem to be true, however, that more labor pains occur in the birth of the first baby than in subsequent ones. A study in Switzerland indicated that an average of almost twice as many uterine contractions were counted for first mothers as for those having subsequent children.

It is generally believed that a woman in her early twenties is less likely to have a difficult labor than an older woman. Nevertheless, many women past forty have given birth for the first time without difficulty. Some women who married late in life have mothered large families in their forties. Actually, a woman of forty who has always kept herself in good physical condition, with proper exercise and a good diet, may have an easier pregnancy and delivery than some twenty-year-olds who have been indifferent to the principles of good health.

Enough is now known about the psychology of labor so that it can be said that the amount of pain you experience in childbirth will have a striking resemblance to the amount you expect to have. If you are filled with foreboding about what the hospital has in store for you and look ahead to labor with dread, your mental attitude will cause you to react to it intensely.

On the other hand, if you consider that you are generally healthy and have properly prepared yourself, and that millions of women go through this experience year after year without feeling any lasting harm, you will be better equipped to bear whatever pain ensues. It is also well to remember that drugs and anesthetics are now available which can minimize or eliminate pain. Some even help to erase your memories so that you will awaken feeling that you have had almost a painless experience.

If you have ever had adverse effects from any type of anesthesia in the past, you should advise the doctor of this fact, in one of your regular prenatal visits, and again in the hospital, so that he will give you a drug you may tolerate better.

As the pains and contractions become more frequent, do not feel that you must cooperate by bearing down unless your doctor encourages you to do so. This extra effort accomplishes nothing except in the second stage, when it may speed the process of birth. Otherwise it merely consumes your energy unnecessarily and makes you tire. Even with anesthesia, the contractions will come normally.

You will remain in a special labor room while labor continues. A nurse will be nearby constantly, and your doctor will visit you frequently to determine what progress you are making. When he observes that the cervix is completely dilated, he may ask you to bear down with your contractions to facilitate the descent of the baby to the pelvic floor. Then you will be transported to the delivery room for the birth.

You will be placed on a table specially equipped for delivery. You will be given firm supports to hold with each hand. As a contraction develops you will hold the handles and bear down as best you can. This process is virtually instinctive.

With each contraction, the baby moves lower and lower in the birth canal. In a few moments his head will begin to emerge. An incision in the outlet of the birth canal, called an episiotomy, will probably be done to prevent tearing of the tissue and to allow more room for the baby. The doctor will ease the baby's head out gently, then his shoulders, then the rest of his body. Just before this, you may be given a slightly greater amount of anesthesia, and you may not be aware of the actual birth process. The umbilical cord, through which the infant has been sustained in the womb, is then severed.

The doctor will make certain that the baby is breathing properly. Generally his cries will indicate this. Gentle suction may be needed to remove mucous from the mouth and throat and some oxygen may also be given to assist the baby's respirations.

With delivery of the baby, the third stage begins. Its work completed, the placenta separates from the uterine wall. Within a few minutes after the baby has emerged, the uterus contracts again and expels the placenta and membranes. There is generally a moderate amount of bleeding from the uterus but it diminishes rapidly as the uterus contracts. An injection may be given to enforce the contraction.

The birth canal is inspected and the episiotomy is repaired. The baby is then completely examined, weighed and measured, and an antibiotic preparation is instilled in his eyes to prevent infection. You will be kept in a special recovery room for about one hour to make sure your condition is stable, and then you will be wheeled back to your room, and placed in bed.

You probably will sleep for several hours. When you awaken, you may be unable to grasp the fact that you are now a mother with a precious baby to nurture and develop. You may re-member the beautiful words of Jesus from the Gospel of St. John: "A woman about to give birth has sorrow, because her hour has come. But when she has brought forth the child, she no longer remembers her anguish for her joy that a man is born into the world."

Save the mother or the child? Frequently non-Catholics and even some misinformed Catholic patients will ask whether, in Catholic hospitals, "the mother will be sacrificed to save the life of the child." Nothing could be more ridiculous.

No one, no matter what his religion, may deliberately murder one human being to save another, under any circumstances. In any Catholic hospital anywhere, the doctor does his utmost to bring both mother and baby through alive. Occasionally a mother will die in childbirth from complications of pregnancy, but you can rest assured that it was through no direct action of any doctor. Statistics of Catholic hospitals regarding maternal deaths are in every way comparable to and often better than those of non-Catholic institutions.

Men who have been practicing obstetrics for thirty and forty years have never run into a situation where there was the faintest question of making a choice between a mother and her baby. Always, the best treatment is directed for the safety of both.

"Foolproof identification" of your baby. Soon after the baby is born, he will be properly identified. There is no likelihood that a mix-up will occur and you will return home with another mother's infant. A nurse makes sure that the baby you get will be your own by placing your fingerprints and the baby's footprints on the same piece of paper in the hospital records. There is no chance that another baby's footprints will be mistaken for your baby's since footprints have the same individuality as fingerprints. Another device is to attach a tape bearing your name to the baby's wrist, or a bead necklace with your name on it may be placed on the baby and not taken off under any circumstances, to prevent the necklace from being put on the wrong baby.

Circumcision for your boy? If your infant is a boy, your doctor may ask whether you wish to have him circumcised. This is a minor surgical procedure in an infant, and requires no anesthesia. It is usually done a day or two before you go home. By excising the tight foreskin about the glans or head of the penis, future problems of irritation and infection can be avoided. The vast majority of boys are circumcised today except when religious beliefs prohibit it or the father of the baby has strong personal convictions on the question. If you have any doubt about having it done, your own doctor's judgment will probably be the best to follow.

Breech and forceps deliveries. In some cases, the baby's head will not emerge first, but rather his legs or buttocks. This is known as a breech delivery. Labor in such cases may be somewhat longer, and the delivery itself may be more complicated than when the head comes first.

A variation of the usual birth process occurs when the doctor uses forceps to help the baby to emerge. He may decide to use them if labor is unduly prolonged or if the baby does not seem to be making adequate progress down the birth canal. There is little reason for you to be concerned about either a breech or forceps delivery, if you have a competent obstetrician.

Caesarean section. Your doctor may decide that is is necessary to deliver your baby by making an incision through the abdominal and uterine walls, rather than risk a vaginal delivery which may be dangerous because of some special condition. There are several reasons for this operation. For instance, your pelvis may be too small or the baby too large for normal passage through the pelvis. In other cases, such as when diabetes or the Rh factor are present, it may be advisable to deliver the infant earlier than normally. Perhaps natural delivery will be either impossible or less safe than delivery through the abdomen.

When a baby is delivered in this way, a Caesarean section is said to have been performed. Many people believe that this operation derives its name from Julius Caesar, who was said to have been born this way. It makes a good story, but historians do not confirm it. In fact, this was an ancient method of delivery before Caesar was born.

In ancient times this procedure was dangerous—every operation was, because men knew little about surgical techniques, about anesthesia or the importance of sanitary conditions. Childbirth itself was a great deal more dangerous because of the same factors.

But Caesarean section is now a routine procedure. It is done several times weekly in many maternity hospitals, and the rate of maternal and infant mortality is almost infinitesimal. In some hospitals, thousands of such operations have been performed with rarely a casualty.

If a woman has had one Caesarean section, it may be necessary that future babies be delivered the same way. The doctor may think that the scar in the uterus from the previous section should not be endangered by the expansion and contraction of normal labor. In such cases, he may ask the patient to go to the hospital a week or two before the baby is due. He may perform the section at that time, or may wait until labor begins before performing it.

The number of children you can safely have by Caesarean section cannot be given in an exact figure, because each case has to be individualized. However, there are some women who have had as many as ten children by this means.

The period of convalescence in the hospital after a Caesarean section may run to ten days or so—about twice as long as after a baby is delivered normally. But after this period, the mother will be able to get around as well as anyone else who has had a baby.

Premature birth. Regardless of the length of your pregnancy, if your baby weighs less than five and a half pounds at birth, he is considered premature, and is treated as such. He will be given special care until he weighs at least five and a half pounds. He may also be considered premature if born two or more weeks before the expected date.

If your baby is exceptionally small at birth, he will probably be placed in an incubator. This is a covered crib with its own source of oxygen and heat and humidity. The temperature can be very carefully regulated, reproducing conditions similar to those in the womb. If the baby is very small, he may be fed through an eye-dropper or a tiny stomach tube. The mother who wishes to feed her baby with her own milk may be taught how to extract it from the breast by hand or by means of a breast pump. Today premature babies are usually not breast-fed but are given special formulas.

The infant will be kept in the incubator until he gains sufficient weight, and the mother may be unable to hold him for several days or weeks. If the infant is very tiny, the baby will undoubtedly have to remain in the premature unit after the mother returns home.

The importance of hospital care for a "premie" cannot be overemphasized. We have made great strides in caring for these tiny infants, and even a baby born several months too early may survive if given the special treatment he needs. A premature baby may take a long time to catch up to full-term infants born on the same date. Eventually, however, he will be just as sturdy as anyone. Incidentally, he will join some distinguished company. Julius Caesar, Isaac Newton and Winston Churchill, among other famous men of history, all were born prematurely. Their early entry into this life did not handicap them in the living of it.

What to do if the baby is born suddenly. Some expectant mothers fear that their babies will be born before they reach the hospital or before a doctor can be called. In almost all cases, an expectant mother has ample time to reach the hospital. It is more likely that you will become impatient at the length of time that labor requires after you are in the hospital.

If the improbable were to happen in your case, however, you might realize that very rapid births almost always happen only in the case of healthy babies, and that if your baby is born before you get to the hospital, he will almost surely be normal. Secondly, you might remember that babies have been born without benefit of doctors for thousands of years and that most of the world's infants are born this way today.

You could have a perfectly normal birth without complications in your own home. The reason doctors insist upon a hospital as a place of birth is that the hospital has the necessary facilities if you or your baby should require special emergency care. They take this precaution to make conditions at your delivery as safe as humanly possible.

Because some mothers are relieved to have instructions to refer to in the highly unlikely event that no medical attendant will be on hand when the baby comes, the following procedures for assisting at childbirth are given.

When labor begins, make sure to call the doctor or an ambulance. Then enlist the assistance of a relative or friend. Lie down in a comfortable place.

If the labor pains are occurring every minute or so, tell your assistant to wash her hands thoroughly with soap and hot water. She should place newspapers under your hips and cover the papers with clean towels upon which the baby will be born.

Let nature take its course. The sac of water surrounding the baby generally will break before he emerges from the birth canal. If the sac is unbroken when the baby appears, it should be pricked with a pin or the tip of a pair of scissors.

Using a clean handkerchief, the helper should wipe the sac and fluid away from the baby's face and head. She should also carefully wipe the mouth and nose.

The baby should now be moved a short distance from the vagina, between your legs. The umbilical cord attached to his navel should not be stretched but should be permitted to remain loose. To be sure that no fluid or secretion runs into his mouth or nose, a small pillow might be used to elevate his head slightly. Make sure that his breathing is normal. Crying is a good sign. It indicates that he is using his lungs.

It will be safe to leave him in this position for an hour or so. By then, the doctor or ambulance will probably have arrived. The doctor or ambulance attendant will be able to sever the umbilical cord and perform the necessary remaining steps.

Simply make sure that the baby is resting in a clean spot, that the umbilical cord has some slack to it, and that his body is covered with a towel or blanket to keep him warm. Do not cover his head, for that might obstruct his breathing.

In the extremely unlikely event that a doctor, ambulance attendant or other medical attendant such as a nurse is not on hand within an hour after birth, it is desirable to cut the umbilical cord. This is not a difficult or complicated task.

Using strong, clean twine or tape, your helper should tightly tie the cord in two places—the first place about six inches from the baby's navel and the second place about eight inches from it. Now she should cut between the two places tied. She should use clean scissors—if possible, a pair which has been sterilized in boiling water and allowed to cool.

After the cord has been cut, your helper can remove the baby from the bed and place him on his side in a warm basket or some other place where he is wrapped warmly but has his face uncovered.

The afterbirth will come by itself, usually a few minutes after the baby is born. You need not take any action to speed it. The umbilical cord will come with the placenta and other expelled matter onto the newspaper. Keep the placenta for the doctor to examine.

Following delivery of the afterbirth, the uterus should be kept firm. It can be felt as a large lump, just below the navel. Your assistant should form a circle around it with her hands and rub it gently until it seems firmly contracted and bleeding slows down. Should it relax and soften, she should again stimulate it by gentle stroking. You can check this yourself.

She might now clean your buttocks and thighs. She should not clean around the vagina, however, as it is wise to avoid the risk of infection at this time.

Now you might have hot tea, coffee or milk if you desire it. Make sure that the baby is warm, safe and comfortable—and relax.

YOUR CARE AFTER BIRTH

When you awaken after giving birth, you may find it difficult at first to grasp the fact that your abdomen is much smaller than it was before. There will probably be a certain amount of soreness—a natural condition in view of the strenuous exercise you have been through—but there should not be severe pain at this time.

Your doctor will probably see you soon after you awaken, and you should tell him if you experience severe pains or have any other difficulties. It is not unusual for new mothers to have trouble urinating. A nurse may easily catheterize you to remedy the situation.

Gradual changes in convalescence. There will be a slight flow from the vagina which may be heavier than a menstrual period. The flow may continue for as long as two or three weeks while the uterus gradually returns to its normal size.

After that time, a whitish discharge may continue. Your doctor will advise you how to handle this condition. He may recommend a douche. If so, he will instruct you how to do this.

Be prepared to spend about six weeks in convalescing from confinement. At the end of that time, you should be close to your normal physical self again and should be able to carry on your regular household duties. During this six weeks, there will be a gradual change in your body. For example, immediately after your baby is born, your uterus will weigh about two pounds. It will steadily diminish in size until it reaches its weight before you became pregnant—about two ounces.

There also will be significant changes in your breasts. Soon after birth, they will secrete a watery but protein-rich fluid which can nourish your baby. Then they will gradually become firmer and fuller and the veins will become more conspicuous. The added weight may cause slight pain, but you can relieve this condition by wearing a firm, well-fitted brassiere which holds them properly.

About the third or fourth day milk will begin to come into the breasts. As long as the baby feeds from them, new milk will be produced. Unless the breasts are regularly emptied of the milk, however, you may experience pain. Therefore you should get instructions from your doctor on how to prevent them from filling up if you do not nurse your baby. He may order pills or injections to restrict production of milk, or may suggest that ice bags be applied to the breasts.

Preparations for breast-feeding. As was mentioned earlier, you should decide before giving birth whether or not to nurse your infant. Unfortunately, no test can determine conclusively in advance whether you will be able to provide enough milk to meet your baby's needs. Neither the size, shape or other characteristics of the breasts seem to make any difference. But it can be said in advance that the mother with a calm, serene attitude generally makes a more efficient nurse than one who is keyed-up and nervous. However, it is also known that moderate exercise in the open air indirectly helps milk production, and that the mother who eats a high proportion of protein foods is likely to have richer milk.

Certain substances which a nursing mother eats will appear almost immediately in her milk. Among these is alcohol. It will appear in the same proportion in the milk as it does in the mother's blood, and if a nursing mother becomes intoxicated, her baby might be adversely affected also. Sedatives will also show up in the milk. Moderate smoking does not seem to affect either the quality or quantity of mother's milk, however.

Breast-feeding and child-spacing. There seems less chance of becoming pregnant again when the mother breast-feeds than when artificial feeding is resorted to. Records of several generations ago seem to substantiate this. A remarkable natural spacing of births by women who practiced breast-feeding but did not resort to artificial contraception can be observed. Their children were usually born two years (more or less) apart. Thus, it may be deduced that additional pregnancies are unlikely while a mother breast-feeds a baby. The evidence suggests, however, that conception becomes increasingly likely after ten or twelve months of breast-feeding.

If you breast-feed your baby, your doctor will recommend a diet which will probably emphasize protein foods—meat, cheese, eggs, milk—as well as daily portions of fresh fruits and vegetables, whole grain and enriched cereals. Probably he will also urge you to drink six to eight glasses of water or other fluids each day.

Recovering your strength. Your doctor will outline what you may do day by day as you gain new vigor after your baby's birth. Modern doctors usually do not insist upon the long period of bed rest immediately after birth that was generally recommended a generation ago. The reason is that mild exercise serves as a general tonic and tends to build strength rather than diminish it.

The first day after delivery, you probably will want to rest a great deal. There is no reason for you to get out of bed except to go to the bathroom. When this is allowed by the doctor, very few patients will have difficulty passing their urine. Many patients find it difficult or impossible to urinate on a bedpan, and may have to be catheterized to prevent overdistention of the bladder.

As the patient is allowed bathroom privileges with assistance, she soon feels stronger and gradually after two or three days is up and about on her own. Frequent, short movements and walks are more desirable than long periods out of bed once or twice a day. Getting out of bed, walking around it once and getting back in bed every one or two hours is an ideal method. Patients often feel so well that they attempt to do too much, and this should be avoided. Rest is necessary but confinement to bed is not. You are usually allowed to guide yourself in your activity. Visitors are a nice change of pace from the hospital routine, but too often patients are exhausted by an endless stream of well-wishers, and this is certainly not to be encouraged.

The date of your discharge from the hospital will depend upon your condition and your doctor's judgment. He will not wish you to remain for either a shorter or longer period than he regards as necessary. When you leave, he will suggest procedures for you at home. He may approve of light housework, provided you rest frequently and do little or no stair-climbing.

While you are in the hospital and for several weeks after your return, you will be urged to take shower baths. Tub baths are generally not recommended until the mouth of the uterus is fully closed, because tub waters might contain bacteria which could cause an infection. It is considered safe to resume tub baths after the discharge from the vagina ceases to show traces of blood.

Exercises to help you regain your figure. Your doctor may recommend exercises to help restore your abdominal muscles and your other organs to normal. Inasmuch as individual circumstances vary a great deal, you should do no exercises immediately after childbirth without his approval. Some physicians believe that special exercises are unnecessary, and that a return to normality can be achieved if you go about your regular activities in a moderate way.

A typical exercise designed to reduce the abdomen consists in lying flat on your back, with arms at your sides, and trying to raise your head and bring your chin to your chest without bracing yourself or moving your legs. Most women require at least several days of exercising before they can do this.

Here are other routines which are often recommended: Lie on your back. Raise one leg as high as possible and bring it back as far to your head as you can. You must not raise your head or bend your knees while doing this exercise.

Lying on your back, bend one knee and pull the leg as close to your body as you can. Repeat with the other leg. After several weeks, you may be able to bring both legs up together.

Any exercises will be difficult to do at first. But if you follow a consistent, daily program—with your doctor's approval— you will surely achieve satisfactory results after a time.

These exercises will help to to redistribute any excess fat you may have gained during pregnancy. When you step on the scales after giving birth, you will probably be at least several pounds heavier than when you became pregnant. In delivery, you will have lost about fourteen pounds. As your organs return to normal, you probably will lose another four pounds. Any excess weight you have two weeks after delivery will have to be lost by exercise, diet or both.

When will you menstruate again? Mothers who do not nurse their babies generally menstruate about six or eight weeks after delivery. Those who nurse may not menstruate again for eighteen months, but it is more likely to be five or six months. Your first few periods may follow a different pattern from that which you knew before you became pregnant, and it may be several months before you again achieve regularity on a predictable basis.

Many women who had cramps and other menstrual discomforts before pregnancy discover that their periods after childbirth are virtually painless. There is an erroneous but widely held belief that you cannot become pregnant until after the first menstrual period. The fact is that your ovaries begin to function shortly after the delivery, preparing an egg for ovulation. The egg can be fertilized by the male sperm when it is mature and extruded before a period can possibly occur.

Your last checkup. Until he discharges you, you should regard yourself as under your obstetrician's care. Even after you return from the hospital, feel free to call him if you experience physical difficulties. The total fee which most obstetricians charge includes post partum care and a final checkup about six weeks after delivery.

At that time, he will ask you to go to his office. He will examine your internal organs, abdomen and breasts. He will take a specimen of urine and check your blood pressure and do a blood count. If he uncovers a condition requiring further treatment, he will inform you of this fact. If he gives you a "clean bill of health," it means that you are now ready to resume your normal activities.

Patients are usually advised to refrain from marital relations until after this examination. If your condition is normal, you may resume your normal sex life.

Facts about the rhythm method. At this final examination, some obstetricians suggest methods of artificial contraception to their patients, and sometimes volunteer to fit the contraceptive devices that they recommend. If you tell your doctor that you are a Catholic and believe that the use of contraceptives is wrong, he will probably drop the matter. If he has an understanding of Catholic teachings, he may aid you by explaining the rhythm method. Catholic doctors will endeavor to explain how it is possible to avoid conception by refraining from intercourse during the short fertile period in every month which is the only time when conception can occur. Here is what you should know about this natural method of family limitation.

First, who may practice the rhythm method? Pope Pius XII set forth these conditions in 1951. While pointing out that married couples have a moral obligation to help conserve the human race, His Holiness declared that at certain times and under certain conditions, natural methods might be employed to excuse a couple from fulfilling this obligation. In other words, the Church does not expect a Catholic mother to go from pregnancy to pregnancy in an endless chain.

His Holiness cited four "indications" which would justify use of the rhythm method. These "indications" are:

Medical reasons. For example, a doctor may advise a mother against having children at some particular time. A woman still recovering from childbirth might be advised to avoid the conception of another child until she fully regains her strength. A woman with a serious and incurable disease might be warned of the strong likelihood of her death and the possibility that her baby would become an orphan. A woman whose husband was in bad health might be justified in practicing periodic continence if their child in all likelihood would face a fatherless future.

Your medical adviser's judgment should be respected. But sometimes it is wise not to accept at face value statements to the effect that a woman's life may be endangered if she becomes pregnant again. Opinions of doctors often differ on this subject. However, you are under no obligation to accept the judgment of one who denies that a serious danger exists. For your own psychological well-being, you probably should seek the opinions of several physicians.

Eugenic reasons. These may exist when a couple is likely to produce defective children or to give them serious diseases, such as epilepsy, a certain type of diabetes, etc.

Economic reasons. If a couple cannot reasonably support a child, they are under no obligations to conceive one. What constitutes "reasonable ability to support a child"? That is something of a question. You need not live in abject poverty—in the poor section of town, without the common comforts of life —before you are justified in practicing the rhythm method on these grounds. On the other hand, you should not feel that economic reasons exist if you would have to forego an extra cocktail before dinner or a new car every other year in order to support a new life.

Social reasons. These might be present if certain conditions made it extremely difficult or impossible for you to have a normal family life. For instance, housing accommodations were difficult to find in America after World War II. Many couples were forced to live with in-laws—perhaps in one room of an apartment or house. Under such circumstances, they might have been excused from having children until they could provide some kind of home of their own.

In a current case, a husband in the armed forces may be required to spend a long tour of duty overseas where he will be unable to have his family with him and will be unable to serve as a father to his children.

In situations when the practice of the rhythm method might be permitted, the Church requires that two additional requirements be met: First, both partners must agree to practice it. A wife may not insist on abstinence during her fertile period if her husband wishes to engage in the act. She may not do so because in the marriage contract, she and her husband both agreed to satisfy the other's reasonable requests for marital relations. The second condition is that both husband and wife must be able to abstain during the fertile period without the danger that either will seek sexual satisfaction through other outlets.

How the rhythm method works. This method is based upon the scientific truth that a woman is fertile only for a short period during the average menstrual cycle. She is sterile—incapable of conceiving—on other days. Obviously, if she has intercourse only on sterile days—and refrains from intercourse on her fertile days—she will not become pregnant.

Your understanding of the way your body was prepared for the birth of your baby will enable you to realize why you are fertile only a short time each month. As was explained in the chapter describing how your baby was conceived, approximately each month the typical woman brings to maturity an egg in either of her two ovaries. Around the middle of her menstrual cycle the egg is discharged from the ovary in the process of ovulation. It enters the abdominal cavity and travels through one of the two Fallopian tubes to the uterus. This movement requires about three days.

This egg must be fertilized if conception is to take place, and this usually occurs in the outer part of the tube. For this to happen, it must be united with the male sperm during its trip to the uterus. If unfertilized during that time, the egg will die. The cycle continues in motion and the lining of the uterus will be disposed of in the next menstrual period.

It is believed that sperm live about one to three days. Sperm deposited in the vagina twenty-four to seventy-two hours before ovulation may be alive and in the tube as the egg travels to the uterus, and may therefore fertilize it. This period, plus the time required for the egg to make its way into the tube, means that conception is likely if intercourse occurs on only about four days in each monthly cycle.

Most young couples could doubtless exercise restraint during four days out of each month. However, exact methods of predicting when these days will occur have not yet been worked out. Physicians therefore recommend that couples avoid intercourse on extra days around the ovulation time.

Two methods of determining the time of ovulation are now in general use. They are:

Basal body-temperature method. There is usually a pronounced rise in body temperature when ovulation occurs. The rise is believed to be related to the fact that the level of the hormone progesterone rises when the egg leaves the ovary. Putting this method to use, a woman might maintain careful body temperature readings and thus pinpoint when ovulation occurs.

A thermal chart must be kept to record temperature variations at different periods of the monthly cycle. A typical chart shows that the body temperature just after menstruation is about a degree lower than what it will be after ovulation. Just before ovulation, there may be a slight dip and then a pronounced rise. When this rise is maintained, it indicates that ovulation has occurred.

If this method is to be used with proper accuracy, records should be kept for about four months in order to determine the patterns that apply in a particular woman's case. During this period, she would take her basal temperature preferably at the same time—before rising each morning—and certainly before breakfast or before she began her day's activities. A special thermometer—one which contains readings in tenths of degrees —is necessary. After examining her records, her doctor could show the woman how to determine her ovulation time by the increase in her temperature and its duration.

The temperature method of determining fertile and sterile periods can be as efficacious as any other form of family limitation. Of course, the need to take regular temperature readings and to keep records makes this method difficult to use. However, it is most accurate when relations are limited to the days after the temperature has been elevated for three mornings, indicating that ovulation has occurred and by that time the ovum is dead.

Fertility testor method. This seems less involved than the other methods. It is based upon the findings of competent researchers that increased amounts of glucose are secreted from the cervix at the time of ovulation.

A special test tape has been developed which changes color

in the presence of this sugar. It therefore becomes a simple matter for the woman to insert a device into the vagina to which this special tape is attached. A few days before the beginning of her fertile period, the tape may start to change color. There is an increased secretion of glucose upon the actual day of ovulation, and the test tape will show a strong reaction. If the married couple refrains from intercourse at the first indication of a color change and for at least a day after ovulation has been signaled, it is unlikely that conception will occur.

These two natural methods of family limitation are morally permissible since they do not create artificial barriers against conception. So-called "birth control" methods do employ artificial means. This may be a device worn by the man or the woman, a douche taken after intercourse to kill the male sperm, or pills which inhibit the hormones necessary for a woman to conceive a child. The use of all such methods is sinful and against nature, and leads to the abuse of the sexual privilege.

Large families are the Christian ideal. A Catholic discussion of the subject of family limitation is incomplete if it does not stress the fact that Christian societies have always upheld the large family as the ideal. In the words of Pope Pius XII, such a family has "been blessed by God, beloved by the Church and considered by it as one of its most precious treasures."

In a memorable address to the Association of Large Families of Rome, His Holiness said that "faith in God supplies parents with the strength necessary to face the sacrifices and the renunciations required for the rearing of children; Christian principles guide and lighten the difficult task of education; the Christian spirit of love watches over the family's order and tranquility while it dispenses, almost drawing upon nature itself, the intimate family joys common to parents, children and brothers." The Pope added:

"But God also visits large families with His Providence, to which the parents, especially poor ones, give an open testimony by placing in it their entire trust, when human efforts are not sufficient. It is a trust well-founded, and not in vain . . . God does not deny the means to live to those He calls to life."

It should also be borne in mind that students of the factors that make for happiness in marriage have come to the almost unanimous conclusion that such happiness is closely associated with "a strong desire to have children." Generally speaking, the least happy marriages are those in which the partners look upon a child as a burden to be avoided.

Disadvantages of the rhythm method. It is difficult to predict ovulation precisely and if abstinence is therefore necessary for more than a few days at a time, the use of the rhythm method may involve drawbacks. Moreover, if you make avoiding conception your all-important goal, you may often find yourself tense and uncertain, fearing that pregnancy may have occurred. Such tensions often cause lasting habits of irritability and resentment-patterns which reflect themselves adversely in other phases of marriage.

If a couple practices periodic continence for long periods, they may find themselves expressing their emotions "by the calendar." On fertile days, they may repress their natural feelings of affection lest the display lead to intercourse. A continued avoidance of such displays may result in a de-emphasis of the spiritual and emotional qualities which should contribute to the act of married love, and may tend to overaccentuate the physical aspects of the act.

If you plan to make use of the rhythm method, it would be well to seek the help and advice of a doctor experienced with its use and with recent advances in the field.

The obstetrician's final advice. If you have been found to be in good condition at your postpartum examination, your doctor will now discharge you. You should, however, return for examinations periodically, perhaps once a year. You should return sooner if any problem related to your reproductive organs arises. As obstetrics is a combined specialty with gynecology, your doctor is the one best equipped to handle any of these problems.

3

Preparing for Your Baby

A. J. VIGNEC, M.D.
Medical Director, New York Foundling Hospital

It is a rare new mother who does not feel some twinges of anxiety over the different experiences she will face in bringing up her baby. There are many plans to be made, many things to be learned. This does not mean, however, that you should feel any deep concern over your ability to perform the tasks of motherhood adequately. Millions of young women have faced this problem of parenthood without the modern opportunity to learn, through reading and other sources, how to care for the baby. If you learn beforehand what must be done and how to do it, you will have the first essential for success as a parent —the confidence and peace of mind that comes from knowing what you are doing.

One of the most important ways of gaining this confidence is to make sure, before your baby is born, that you will always be able to turn to a competent pediatrician—a physician who specializes in the medical care of children. Therefore, select a "baby doctor" in advance. Like obstetricians, pediatricians can be found in most medium-sized and large communities. Perhaps the doctor who is now taking care of you will recommend a pediatrician. If he is a general practitioner, he might care for the baby too.

You might use the same methods to find a baby doctor as

you did in getting a doctor to care for you during your pregnancy. The local County or State Medical Society may give you the names of several accredited pediatricians in your community. You might even inquire at a reputable hospital for the names of such doctors on its staff. If the hospital is highly regarded, you can be confident that the pediatricians accredited to it will likewise be first-rate.

You probably should arrange to see the pediatrician a month or so before your baby is expected, in order to discuss questions about feeding he will later have to supervise. If you intend to breast-feed your baby, this is a decision that should be made early. The pediatrician may have definite ideas he will want you to follow. In any event, he will want you to prepare yourself for all that this type of nursing entails. He may or may not visit the baby in the hospital, but he should have the infant under his care when you return home.

If you cannot afford a pediatrician in private practice, your local hospitals or community welfare agency can probably refer you to a free clinic where you can bring your baby for a regular examination. In rural areas, there may be a State Health Department with visiting nurses who will call on you periodically to see that all is well with your baby, and refer you to a clinic if immediate medical care is indicated.

You will doubtless be besieged with advice from well-meaning friends and relatives about the care of your baby. In fact, you may get so much conflicting information that you will become confused. You might do well to decide at the outset to pay careful attention to your pediatrician and perhaps to one or two others who are doing a good job of caring for their own babies. Accept with thanks, and with many grains of salt, the advice you may get from others.

Layette arrangements. Some months before the expected birthdate, you should accumulate the things you will need to care for your baby when you return from the hospital. If you wait, you may find yourself pressed for time in the last month. If you list the items you will need and shop for them at leisure, you will probably get better quality goods at lower prices than if you rush out to buy everything at once.

You do not need very much. Some mothers buy too much in a burst of enthusiasm, then discover how few things they really needed. Your baby will not mind if you do not get the most expensive items available.

You will need a place for him to sleep—a bed with sturdy sides to keep him from falling out, and with a soft, firm mattress. During the first month or so, the bed might be an oversized clothes basket. The mattress should be made to fit the crib; occasionally an old blanket folded several times may temporarily serve the purpose.

Modern mothers use waterproof sheets which can be put into the washing machine or into boiling water. If these are not available, a piece of plain rubber sheeting is adequate. *Never, never* use the fine thin plastic which is used by dry cleaners and many manufacturers to cover their products. This substance is highly dangerous, as it clings to the baby's skin, shutting out oxygen and at times causing strangulation.

The rubber or other waterproof sheeting is designed to protect the mattress from urine stains. It should be covered by a regular white cotton sheet (preferably knitted), fitted to the size of the mattress or large enough to tuck in under the sides. Most mothers use a soft absorbent pad, quilted or made of heavy Turkish toweling, to put directly under the baby. These are comfortable, easily laundered, and often keep the sheet dry as well. Usually, four to six such pads are required. The sheets are usually changed once a day. If you intend to wash every other day, four sheets should be sufficient, allowing for drying time. If you ever lack clean sheets, sterilized diapers may serve in an emergency. Several diapers would be needed of course, so that they would overlap.

Several light-weight blankets will probably suffice. By using light blankets, you will be able to increase or reduce the number depending upon temperature conditions in the house. Wool or orlon blankets provide maximum warmth for their weight. Orlon is more practical, since washing is easier and there is less shrinkage.

Small cotton blankets, commonly called "receiving blankets," are very useful to wrap a small baby in. This is done at many hospitals, and often mothers continue the practice at home. These small square blankets are quite reasonably priced.

Clothing for the baby need not be expensive. The following is probably all that you will need:

Four to six cotton shirts, size two. These will be slightly large for a newborn baby but will just fit him after a few months. Shirts that are reinforced at the point where they are pinned to the diaper are often recommended, for they have a longer life. Include several long-sleeved shirts if you live in a cold climate, or if the baby is born in late summer or autumn.

Four cotton nightgowns or kimonos. Some long nightgowns have a string running through the bottom hem, which you can tie for extra warmth. These gowns are made with a full cut. The baby can exercise his legs without feeling any restriction.

Two washable sweaters of different weights—one for moderately cool temperatures, the other for colder weather.

A *lined bunting* to be worn outdoors if it is winter.

Four dozen diapers if you plan to wash them yourself, one dozen if you intend to use a "diaper service." This laundry service is a great boon to some mothers. The diaper firm provides a stated quantity of fresh sterilized diapers each week and carries off those the baby has soiled. A new baby uses a considerable number of diapers, and you may welcome the opportunity to be freed of the necessity of washing diapers several times a week in addition to your other duties.

Some new mothers prefer to save money on entertainment or other things and use it for a diaper service during the early months. However, if you have an automatic washer, diaper laundering need not be a great chore. The diapers have little or no odor if soaked in a pail of water to which a small quantity of borax has been added.

Even if you have a diaper service, you should own a small supply of diapers for emergencies. You can use them as bed or carriage sheets and bibs, or as spares if your baby requires more during a given period than you have received from the service. Buy diapers which are not excessively bulky, and which have a soft texture but good absorbing qualities, and are quick-drying. Diapers are useful for many quick clean-up jobs as well.

Several plastic diapers with disposable pads, for use when you take the baby out. These absorb easily, but may cause a chapped condition if they are not replaced frequently. Loose-fitting pants are generally recommended to insure good circulation and help prevent diaper rash.

Two pairs of short socks to keep the baby's feet warm if you take him out during cold weather. Shoes or bootees are not necessary at this stage.

Equipment for the baby's bath. A table with built-in tub is commonly used, but it is not absolutely necessary. You can use a large pan just as well—even the kitchen sink if it has been carefully scoured ahead of time. Near the place where you intend to bathe the baby, you might keep a supply of sterilized absorbent cotton, sterile gauze pads, a dish containing mild soap, several large safety pins (closed and beyond the baby's reach), a soft washcloth, and other items—such as rubbing alcohol or antiseptic ointment—which the doctor may advise you to use.

Although not essential, a thermometer is used by many mothers to make sure that the temperature of the bath water is about 95 degrees—neither too hot nor too cold. Other mothers say that they gauge the temperature satisfactorily simply by testing the water with their elbow or wrist.

You should have one extra-large bath towel to place on the table or on your lap, on which you can deposit the baby after his bath, and a smaller towel to use in drying him.

Other equipment. Not all parents consider the following articles necessary, but you may find them useful to have, depending on your own circumstances:

Baby carriage. City dwellers use this more than do those who live in the suburbs or the country. A baby carriage should be balanced so that it will not sway or tip over easily. It should have handles that enable you to push without stretching or bending and it should be large enough to fit your baby comfortably throughout his first two years.

Baby scale. This may not be necessary unless your doctor wishes you to maintain a record of the baby's weight. He probably will weigh your baby during each visit and will tell you whether the infant is making satisfactory progress.

Dressing table or bathinette. One which might be used in the bathroom will be a convenience. Some tables have compartments in which you can place soap, baby powders and other essentials.

Other articles for the baby—playpen, high chair, toilet seat, etc.—need not be bought before birth, or even during the first few months. You may be able to borrow them from friends or relatives who do not need them at the moment. If you would prefer to have your own, you might suggest them to friends who ask you what they can get for the baby. If you buy them yourself, do not overlook opportunities to purchase them secondhand from parents who no longer need them.

Feeding supplies. If you do not plan to breast-feed your infant, you will need bottles and sterilizing equipment for making the formula. Even if you breast-feed, you will need such equipment for emergencies—in case you become ill, or for supplemental feedings. You will need:

About a dozen round or rectangular bottles. These must be heat-resistant because they have to be thoroughly sterilized by steaming before each feeding.

Three four-ounce bottles to be used for water, juice, or small formula feedings. These must also be heat-resistant.

Sterilizer and rack. These are specially made to hold formula bottles, and are a great convenience. Some electric units can be plugged in anywhere in the house. A less expensive type, designed to be used on gas or electric ranges, is often preferred because all of the work of preparing the formula generally takes place in the kitchen anyway.

A dozen nipples. These should be a good brand, made to fit over the bottles.

Nine or ten nipple covers. After the formula is made and sterile nipples are placed over the bottles, these caps should be used to keep the nipples sterile until the baby feeds. Some mothers cover the bottles with screw-on caps and leave the sterile nipples in the nipple jar until feeding time.

Nipple jar, with cover, that will hold extra nipples until ready for use. The cover should have small holes to insure thorough steaming. The jar itself should be washed and cleaned, then sterilized with all the other equipment. In addition, you will need a can-opener; a funnel to enable you to pour the formula into the bottles; a long brush to clean the bottles; and a wire-haired brush for nipples. Tongs are useful to lift the bottles out of the sterilizer; and you will need a quart measure with ounce markings so that you will be able to measure the ingredients going into the formula. All the equipment above must be sterilized with the bottles and nipples.

Arranging for household help. At least a month before the baby's due date, you should arrange to have help with your housework after you return from the hospital. If you can, try to sign up someone to "live in" for two or three weeks, handle normal housekeeping routines, do the necessary shopping, prepare meals and the formula, wash clothes, and so on. Then you will be free to care for your baby while obtaining the extra rest you will need to complete your convalescence.

In many communities, practical nurses or trained housekeepers specialize in doing just this kind of work. If your means permit, you might wish to hire one. Your friends, the hospital, the local social service agency, your pastor, may all be able to recommend someone. Women doing such work are generally in great demand and often schedule their assignments many months ahead. Therefore, if you decide to employ outside help, you would do well to make such arrangements as early as you can.

Relatives or friends may volunteer to help you during this time. Before accepting the offers of anyone, make sure it is a person with whom you get along well. *Avoid the "bossy" type who will insist on taking complete charge.* After giving birth, you will be in a condition which unfortunately lends itself to misunderstandings and disagreements over who should do what and who should make the decisions. You will not be well enough to do many jobs yourself, but you will be well enough to have firm ideas about how they should be done. If you have a domineering relative or friend in your house, you may find yourself impatiently waiting for her to leave.

The same potential difficulty may apply if you have a paid houseworker. Try to make sure in advance that her personality will not conflict with your own. Ask her to give names of women she has worked for and ask them about her qualifications and disposition.

Precautions to take if you "go it alone." Of course, many mothers have survived without outside help. If you must go it alone for financial or other reasons, make two resolutions:

First, that for one month, you will do only what is absolutely necessary. You will perhaps be surprised at how much dusting, mending, cleaning, and other chores you can avoid if you turn your eyes from them. Have the simplest meals for yourself and your husband—perhaps packaged foods which need only to be thawed or taken from a can and heated.

Second, that you will try to get your husband to help as much as possible. In many areas, food stores remain open at least one evening a week, and he may be able to do the family's grocery shopping. If you lack an automatic clothes washer, he might take the dirty clothes to a "laundromat" or a quick-service laundry. He can learn to sterilize the feeding equipment and bottles, prepare a day's supply of formula each evening, and even give the baby his daily bath.

How long will it be before you can do these jobs yourself? Naturally, the answer will depend upon how well you have prepared yourself to care for a baby and how quickly you regain your strength. Generally, new mothers should have outside help for two or three weeks. Another two or three weeks should elapse before they do all the household tasks they did before.

Incidentally, you and your husband should face the prospect that with a small baby to care for, you will no longer be able to keep your home as spic and span as it was before you became pregnant. You will have to leave some household jobs undone so as to give your baby the care and attention he deserves. This is as it should be. Your first job is that of wife and mother—one who will give personal attention to her loved ones.

Babies have grown to happy childhood and good, responsible adulthood in homes where furniture needed dusting and did not get it. But it is much harder for them to become normal, well-adjusted adults if they constantly fail to receive the love and affection they need because Mother is always "too busy with housework."

Getting to know your baby. You will doubtless be astonished when you see your baby for the first time. Unless you have seen many newborn infants before, you may even be disappointed. He will probably be smaller, redder and generally a great deal different from the image of an infant that flashed into your mind when you heard the word "baby" in the past.

The average newborn infant weighs about seven and a half pounds. The majority vary in weight from five to eleven pounds. The usual length is about twenty inches—little more than one and a half feet.

At birth, he will have an agreeable fragrance all his own—one you will perhaps never forget. This is due to the fact that at birth, a white substance known as "vernix" covers his skin and serves as a protective coating.

In many ways, he is still not completely formed. His head may be slightly out of shape due to the pressure exerted upon it as it traveled through the pelvic canal. However, baby bones are soft and flexible and regain their former shape after a few days. There will be a soft spot in the center of the scalp. This spot—the "fontanelle"—will close gradually over a period of several months. By then, the fine soft fuzz covering his head will be gone, and in its place will be recognizable human hair.

Your baby's body will be small in proportion to his head. His legs will be bowed and will, of course, show no evidence of the muscles he will later develop. He will be toothless. His eyes will roll about aimlessly, and they will not begin to focus and see clearly for perhaps two months.

He will display one primitive instinct—hunger—and will let you know plainly and unmistakably when he wants food. He may or may not cry if he is wet. His nervous system is likely to be sensitive to sharp, sudden noises, and he is likely to cry if he hears one. It will probably take at least several weeks before he indicates even slight awareness of what is going on around him, and it may be a few months before he learns to smile or greet you with recognition.

In addition to food and warmth, he will need to be held, cuddled and loved. He has spent nine months in your womb in complete security, sheltered from all the conditions of our world. When he was born, he was abruptly taken out of his warm, comfortable home. It is natural that he should feel insecure. But some of his sense of security can be restored if you often hold him close to you, letting him feel your heartbeat as he felt it in your uterus, and also the protecting warmth of your body. Babies can survive many deprivations. But they suffer most if they are deprived of what even a poverty-stricken mother can give—the sense of love, protection and security.

That is why pediatricians and child-care specialists emphasize that how you feed your baby is important to his emotional development. In breast-feeding, of course, you must hold him close to you. But the bottle-fed infant should also be held close. Regardless of what other work remains undone, always give him that comforting personal attention.

During his first weeks of life, you will come to understand his language to a surprising extent. For example, you may learn to distinguish different meanings in the different ways he cries. Some mothers can detect one note of urgency if the baby is hungry, another note if he is wet, perhaps a third if indigestion bothers him. You will also learn when your baby should stop crying—for example, after a regular feeding—and you will learn to look for causes other than hunger if he cries at odd hours. Perhaps most important of all, you will recognize that a cry that is not immediately answered may not necessarily lead to tragedy. Soon you should be able to accept his cries as a request that something be done for him, but you will not be failing in your duties if you do not respond to the first wail.

Learning to breast-feed. If you expect to nurse your baby, you will have to be ready to spend several days and perhaps endure some frustrating moments before you and the baby make the system work. After a few difficulties, some mothers give up and decide to use a formula. If they gave the breast-feeding system a little more time, they and their babies might have mastered the art of it.

Your baby must learn to suck effectively, so that he can draw nourishment from your breast. Sucking is a natural instinct, and a normal baby will learn how to do it within a few days. Doctors have found that a baby learns faster if he is spurred by hunger. For that reason, some withhold a bottle feeding if the infant at first does not get the nourishment he needs from the breast.

Your first attempt at breast-feeding probably will not take place until the baby is at least twelve hours old. He will probably not get much milk at this time, but both the supply and his ability to extract it should increase in subsequent feedings.

Your doctor may suggest that you feed your baby regularly every three or four hours. Or he may advise you to let the infant set his own schedule. This means that you will feed "on demand"—when he announces he is hungry, whether one hour or six hours have elapsed since the last feeding. The "self-demand" method has in its favor the fact that the baby eats when he is hungry, not when the clock says he should be fed. On the other hand, it may not always prove practicable to feed your baby when he wants his milk—for example, when you are traveling.

You may need guidance in learning how to breast-feed. As noted above, sucking is a natural instinct. If you direct your infant's mouth to the nipple, he will soon begin sucking. As his efforts produce results, he will continue and intensify them to get the food he wants. After a few days, he will go to the breast as a matter of course. Later he may even reach for it himself.

At first, he may not get enough from one breast to satisfy his hunger. You might then move him to the other. Do not interfere with his breathing as he sucks.

You may have to hold the top of your breast to prevent it from obstructing the passage of air to his nose. If he cannot breathe through his nose, he will try to swallow air. As a result, he may get a great deal of air into his stomach.

In order to give him an opportunity to remove air, rest his head on your shoulder after the feeding. Support his head with one arm, and his back with the other. If you pat his back gently, he will probably belch. Keep a diaper over your shoulder, because he may spit up some milk as he does so.

To keep your nipples soft and clean, you might wash them with soap and warm water after each feeding, or at least wipe them. Some mothers wipe off excess milk after each feeding and thoroughly wash the nipples in their daily bath or shower. If the nipples become sore or begin to crack, your doctor may recommend anointing them with cold cream after each feeding. The cold cream should be washed off thoroughly before the next feeding.

Basic principles of formula-feeding. If you cannot breast-feed your baby or do not wish to do so, your doctor will recommend a formula which will closely approximate your own milk and will contain the food elements the infant needs. Many millions of men and women in good health today were "bottle babies" and there is no medical evidence to suggest that their health is worse than that of men and women who were breast-fed in infancy.

What should be avoided is the tendency to depersonalize the bottle feeding. As in breast-feeding, it should bring mother and child together in order to give him the sense of security and love he needs for good emotional development. If your baby is on a formula, try to make it your rule always to hold him in your arms when feeding him. Avoid the temptation to prop the bottle on a pillow, so that he can suck on it while lying in his crib.

If you cannot hold the baby while he feeds, get your husband, a relative or friend to do so. Many fathers enjoy giving the baby his bottle. They experience some of the satisfactions a mother knows when she holds the baby in her own arms.

If you plan to use a formula, you can learn how to make it, and how to handle the sterilizing equipment, by attending a class for prospective parents. These are held in many hospitals and communities. Your obstetrician or pediatrician can tell you whether such classes are held in your area. If you and your husband attend a course together, you will be thoroughly ready for your job when the baby arrives.

You might also learn how to prepare the formula by carefully following the directions given by the doctor or hospital nurse, or by watching a relative or friend who has some personal experience. If your area has a visiting nurse service, you might also arrange to have one call and explain the exact step-by-step process involved.

You might use one of these means to learn how to change, bathe, and dress the baby. Or you might watch a relative or friend with a small baby, carefully noting the step-by-step procedure. A visiting nurse may arrange to come to your home to show you how to bathe a baby.

While the bath procedure is not complicated, there are several important points you must keep in mind. You must keep the water at a temperature of about 95 degrees, so that it is neither too hot nor too cold. You must hold the baby's head firmly so that it does not go below the water. You must always dry him in a safe place, with all bottles, safety pins and other items away from his reach. The nurse can explain how to clean the baby's organs and how to make sure that you do so safely and competently.

You can find out whether a visiting nurse service is available in your community by calling your local Department of Health.

Confidence comes with knowledge. Probably the best way a new mother can develop confidence in her ability to care for her baby is to prepare herself by reading, attending a course in parenthood, and watching how experienced mothers handle their children. If you have this thorough preparation, your sense of confidence will enable you to enjoy your baby as you should.

Ill-prepared parents often are tense and nervous when the baby comes home, and every minor difficulty becomes a major crisis. For example, they may worry frantically when they notice that the breast of their infant—whether a boy or girl—becomes hard and perhaps secretes a fluid like that from the mother's breast. Had they prepared themselves, they probably would have learned in advance that this condition is very normal. It results from a temporary excess of the very hormones which encourage the development of the milk in the mother's breast. The swelling generally disappears after a week or so.

Mothers should also know that normal baby girls sometimes emit a small amount of blood from the vagina. Unless you had learned to expect it, you might be alarmed at the light color and soft consistency of your baby's bowel movements, as well as their frequency.

Probably the best aid to your self-confidence is the realization that you have a doctor you trust and who can be reached at any time to answer your questions. If you have a telephone in your home, or within easy access, you will not be more than a few minutes away from him and will be able to reach him in an emergency. Even if he goes away for a weekend, his telephone-answering service probably will refer you to a doctor who will substitute for him. You should never feel that you are imposing upon the pediatrician if you are troubled by a condition affecting your baby and need his advice.

If you trust in your own good basic common sense, have prepared yourself well for the task of caring for your baby, and realize that you can always call upon a competent doctor at any time of day or night, you can be fully confident of your ability to be a successful mother. With the spirit of relaxation which comes with such confidence, you will be better able to enjoy your baby and also better able to establish a bond of mutual love that will last for the rest of your lives.

4

How to Maintain a Cheerful Attitude

ROBERT P. ODENWALD, M.D.

Former Professor at Catholic University, Washington
Author of Your Child's World

Most expectant mothers probably have some doubts during pregnancy—doubts of their ability to carry a child, doubts that he will be normal, doubts that he will be as intelligent and good-looking as they would like him to be, possibly doubts of their ability to give the guidance he or she needs to grow into useful, happy manhood or womanhood.

As in the case of most other doubts, these can be dispelled by knowledge. The chances are overwhelming that you will give birth to a normal, happy baby. If you have placed yourself under a doctor's care and have arranged to have your baby in a hospital, you have taken the necessary steps to make all the resources of modern medicine available to help you. These resources are formidable. X-ray machines, fluoroscopes, antibiotics, anesthetics, oxygen equipment—all can be used, if necessary, to insure the safety of you and your infant.

If doubts enter your mind, or you experience vague fears about the future, try to pin down their cause. As often as not, you will probably realize that they have no reasonable basis in fact. At this time, it is helpful if you know your own personality.

You may be the worrying type or the shy and anxious type; knowing this, you may be able to make allowances for your reactions to pregnancy.

If something continues to cause you concern, feel free to consult your doctor. Most likely, he will be able to explain that your fears are exaggerated. In any event, you will give him the opportunity to do something about them.

One evening, a pregnant woman turned on the light switch in her living room. There was a flash, caused by a short circuit in the wiring system. The woman threw her hands to her face in a protective reaction. An old neighbor who was visiting her screamed that she should not have done this, for her baby would now have a birthmark for life.

The pregnant woman suspected that this was just another old wives' tale that had come down through the centuries but which has no basis in fact. Nevertheless, the old woman's words had planted a seed. The expectant mother began to think more of what had happened, and began to be certain that her unborn child would be seriously affected.

Fortunately she had the good sense to mention the incident to the doctor on her next visit. He explained that there is absolutely no scientific support for the belief that a baby can be "marked" in such a way. In fact, an infant's "markings" have no relationship to any act by the mother before or during pregnancy.

Probably the best way to fight your fears is to train your mind to turn from unpleasant thoughts and to concentrate on things of positive value instead. For instance, you might tell yourself: "These fears are foolish. Therefore I will not consider them." If you develop an abiding faith in the goodness of God, you will be particularly well equipped to cope with the inevitable tendencies toward depression which may arise during pregnancy. Resign yourself to His plan for you by putting into practice the words of the Lord's Prayer—"Thy Will Be Done."

It is also important to remember that concerns in pregnancy are quite normal. They often stem from the fact that this is a new experience. After you have gone through pregnancy and given birth once, you will not feel such a sense of trepidation. For the mother of a few children, the idea of pregnancy causes but a tiny fraction of the concern which is customary for the first-time mother who has not had such an experience before.

The best way to overcome your doubts about your ability to do a good job as a mother is to find out as much as you can about your baby's physical, spiritual and emotional care. It will convince you that other persons, very much like yourself, have been highly successful mothers. If possible, attend classes for expectant fathers and mothers which may be sponsored by a local hospital or community organization. Your doctor, or the supervisor of the maternity hospital where you expect to give birth, can tell you whether such classes are available in your community. In gaining knowledge, you will also gain confidence for your task ahead. You will have the information you need to help dispel any vague, unreasoning fears that you may have.

The positive approach to maternity. Many of your psychological reactions to pregnancy will depend upon your own feelings about becoming a mother. Some women look forward to it eagerly. They recognize that they can achieve their own fulfillment only in this way, and that they are participating in one of the great works in the world.

If you can keep before you the idea of the great opportunities of motherhood which Monsignor Kelly has described, you will bear any physical discomforts with greater equanimity. On the other hand, a woman who is indifferent to the ideals of motherhood or resents the fact that she is pregnant will doubtless find that every physical difficulty will be magnified—a slight twinge will become a severe pain and a minor discomfort will become a major complication. A feeling that the baby will take something from the mother, rather than adding to her life, makes pregnancy a more difficult time from both the psychological and physical point of view.

Obviously, your ways of thinking which have been developed during your lifetime cannot be undone in a few months. But regardless of your past feelings about pregnancy, try to look upon it in a positive way—as a necessary part of one of the most creative acts of your life, in which you are giving the precious gift of life to another human being. You might reflect that it is opening the way to great spiritual experiences for you. That you will find in it dimensions of love which you never knew were possible. And that the vast majority of mothers are indeed grateful for their children; if permitted to relive their lives, they would undeniably choose to have more children rather than fewer.

Some women who upset themselves with thoughts that they will be unable to carry their baby to full term, or will somehow fail as parents, are perfectionists. They are unable to gain satisfaction from any action which is even slightly less than perfect. They hope to have a "model" child and they expect to raise him in a "model" way. While this is a laudable ambition, it fails to consider the human factor. The truth is that all of us probably fail to achieve our potentialities to the fullest possible extent, and that we are doing well if we achieve even a substantial part of them.

Nobody expects you to have a perfect child or to be a perfect mother. The mathematics of the situation indicate that you will have a normal child—one who is neither the brightest boy nor girl, nor the least gifted with intellect. Given that normal child, you need only exercise a reasonable care as an expectant mother, reasonably follow your doctor's suggestions, and observe reasonable rules of health. No one can criticize you for not doing more than that.

The woman who is dissatisfied when she achieves anything less than perfection often exercises this trait in bringing up her children. But perfectionism almost always fails to achieve the effect intended. The child who comes to believe that he is never permitted to make mistakes—in everyday situations, is not allowed to dirty his clothes, mess up his room, or show bad manners—will eventually realize that he cannot possibly live up to the standards set for him. Too many children have needed psychiatric care because of the unreasonable demands of their perfectionistic parents to permit me to skip over this subject lightly.

Of course, the other extreme is equally undesirable. The expectant mother who decides that she need observe no precautions to insure her welfare and that of her baby is seriously mistaken. However, the woman who goes through her pregnancy with indifference is extremely rare. For every hundred who might be seriously concerned that they are not doing all that they could, there is probably only one who does not care whether she is doing what she should. As far as you personally are concerned, the fact that you are reading this book indicates your desire to insure a successful pregnancy. And if you follow the advice in these pages, there is no likelihood that you could be considered as negligent.

It is also important to realize that what is "normal" in pregnancy covers a wide range. At one extreme is a woman who may have a complex of minor physical symptoms early—even a few weeks after conception, she may experience nausea, headaches, abdominal discomforts. At the other extreme may be the woman who knows no physical changes during the early few months and may even find it difficult to believe that she is pregnant. Between these extremes are probably the majority of expectant mothers—those who have some discomforts.

The woman with a large number of symptoms may be tempted to indulge in a wave of self-pity. If the first few months of pregnancy are like this, she may reason, what will the last months be like?

At the other extreme, the woman without discomfort may actually feel somewhat guilty. Or she may become alarmed that her baby is not developing as he should. Otherwise, wouldn't she have the discomforts she has come to believe are inevitable?

Of course, both of these attitudes are mistaken. The woman who has a difficult time physically is mistaken in thinking that the entire nine months will be like this, because experience teaches that nausea and other complaints generally disappear after the first few months. The woman without discomfort is mistaken, because millions of mothers can testify that you need not spend nine months in suffering as the price for a baby.

If you can see yourself near either of these two extremes, or if you find yourself worried because your symptoms fall somewhere in the middle, your best reassurance can come from your doctor. From the many cases he has handled in the past, he knows what is normal and reasonable to expect. If he tells you your physical reactions are normal, take his word for it. He knows better than you.

Beware of well-meaning friends. Along about the sixth month, a new set of circumstances may affect your thinking. Until now, you may have found it difficult to believe that a living baby was actually developing within you. Now, however, he begins to move about. And as you experience this strange sensation within your womb, the fact that you are going to become a mother takes on a dramatic new meaning.

At this stage, most expectant mothers—particularly first time mothers—spend much time speculating about the child— whether they will have a boy or girl, whether it will be large or small, whether it will have its mother's features or its father's. You may have to take a firm grip on yourself to realize that mothers have often worried needlessly about their baby's possible defects or shortcomings. And then they gave birth to normal babies that were a source of pride and joy to all. Imagining what your baby might be like is fruitless in any event —but particularly so if you let your mind dwell on depressing or pessimistic possibilities.

As your pregnancy becomes obvious, your friends and relatives may begin to regale you with tales of their own experiences in childbirth. Some may delight in talking about their difficulties. Others may feel obliged to repeat every strange, hair-raising tale about pregnancy they have heard of. Because a re-telling of the actual events might not be sufficiently dramatic, they invariably succumb to the human temptation to make the story more gruesome than it really was. If you find yourself listening to such tales—and worse, believing them—remember that normal pregnancies usually do not get talked about. Only the unusual one makes news—and the fact that there are hundreds of normal cases for every unusual one generally goes unmentioned.

Sometimes ideas of what will happen to the baby after birth prey upon an expectant mother's mind. One woman seemed obsessed by fears that her infant would smother. This is an extremely rare occurrence—so rare, in fact, that it causes widespread comment whenever it occurs. However, when she was at an impressionable age, this young woman had heard such stories, and she was convinced that she would have to keep a constant vigil to insure her baby's survival. Although the infant would not be born for several months, she worked herself into a distraught state over this remote possibility.

When she finally became wise enough to ask her doctor about it, he explained that the average baby can safely sleep in any position, and that there is little reason to be concerned about his smothering. He told her that she could put her baby in his crib and cover his body with light blankets without danger. The woman's fears vanished. This case again emphasizes a key point to give you peace of mind: If anything disturbs you, take steps to learn the true facts.

The "shame" of being pregnant. Sometimes one encounters expectant mothers who manifest shame over their condition. For instance, they may be unwilling to appear in public after the fifth or sixth month, when their pregnancy is apparent.

An objection to being stared at is quite normal. However, it is not normal to feel guilty. Those who stare at you—or worse, give any indication that your condition deserves anything but respect—deserve pity, not you.

The belief that pregnancy is "not nice" undoubtedly stems from the puritanical idea that the marital act is inherently evil. We can realize how wrong this belief is when we consider that this is the means God devised to perpetuate the human race, and that Our Lord Himself, the Blessed Virgin and all the saints developed in the womb before birth. Thus you have nothing to be ashamed of in your condition. Rather, you should feel pride that God has chosen you to participate with Him in creating a human being with the potentialities of sainthood.

Akin to the reluctance to appear pregnant in public is the desire to avoid being seen by those persons before whom you have always maintained a chic, fashionable appearance. True, the figure of a woman who will give birth within a few months is not as attractive in the world's eyes as that of a slender, non-pregnant woman, and dressmakers spend less time in creating designs for expectant mothers than they do on designs for other women. Nevertheless, many attractive garments are available. In any event, there is no reason to feel that you must win a fashion show. You did not conceive your child to win a beauty contest.

Most people make all allowances for a pregnant woman. Your intelligent friends will realize fully that the work in which you are now engaged is well worth the risk of being temporarily "unfashionable." Many are the fashionably dressed, immaculately turned-out women who desperately desire a baby but are unable to have one. It is no exaggeration that the greatest emotion an expectant mother generates is that of envy.

Your relations with your husband. A few words might be said here about the relationship between husband and wife during pregnancy. Of course, husbands should try to be particularly considerate during this period. If possible, a husband should strive to relieve his wife of heavy work, as well as of tedious jobs which might tire her unduly and affect her mental outlook. He should try to be a positive force—to reassure her, to calm her if she is upset, to urge her to see her doctor if some symptoms disturb her.

A husband also should try to bring a pleasant attitude into the home. If his wife is alone all day, she looks forward to a cheerful evening with her husband. She needs to be uplifted, rather than depressed with tales of the unhappy events of the day. One young man returned home each night with new reports of his troubles on his job. He made it obvious that his chances of holding it were very slight. Although he did not intend to do so, he created a strong fear in his young wife's mind that he would be unemployed when the baby came and would be unable to support them. She had visions of being turned into the street, her infant in her arms.

It generally is not fully understood that an expectant father may also have fears about his role when the baby is born. He will have the obligation of contributing to the child's support, perhaps for as long as twenty-one years. He will also be required to display moral, emotional, mental and physical leadership so that his child may successfully cope with the problems of growing up. Some prospective fathers develop doubts about their ability to do these things. Such doubts may affect them even more than they affect a prospective mother, because the latter can at least discuss them with her doctor. Frequently, the husband has no one to turn to, and feels it unmanly to reveal his inner fears.

So strive to be cheerful for your husband's sake, as well as your own. Get adequate rest and exercise during the day, so that you will be a cheerful companion in the evening. If you can arrange your schedule to permit it, take a nap in the afternoon. Try to accent the positive—discuss your pleasant experiences during the day more than you discuss your unpleasant ones. Try to avoid subjects which you know from experience may produce arguments. Try to make yourself especially attractive, to be neatly dressed with your hair well groomed. During pregnancy, a woman needs more beauty care than at other times—for her own morale as well.

The happiest husbands-in-waiting seem to be those who can make a direct contribution during the period of pregnancy and who are not forced to play an entirely passive role. For instance, a husband who is handy with tools may prepare the room which will be the child's nursery. He might install easy-to-wash floor tile or make the chests of drawers, bath table and other furniture which will be used in the room.

There will be permanent changes in your relations with your husband after your return from the hospital with the baby. The baby should unify—not divide—his parents. Always make it plain that the baby is his as well as yours, and that you do not intend to let the newcomer usurp any of the affection you previously bestowed upon your husband.

This point requires emphasis because some mothers or fathers devote too much attention to the new baby at the expense of their partner. They fail to display as much affection and interest as they did before, so that the other partner may come to feel "out of it." The baby then unwittingly becomes a competitor.

You can make sure that your husband feels that his own sense of importance is not minimized if you encourage him to enjoy the baby with you. If possible, ask him to give the baby his bath occasionally, to change diapers, to prepare the formula and also to feed the baby sometimes—perhaps at night so that you can have an undisturbed sleep. Encourage him to help make decisions about the baby's care—perhaps the type of furniture to buy. Even if it is not possible for him to help care for the baby physically, make a point of discussing the infant's development with him so that he will never consider himself an unnecessary outsider who disturbs your relationship with the new member of the family.

It is also important to avoid spending so much time in caring for the baby that you cannot do at least some of the things with your husband that you did before you were pregnant. Soon after your return from the hospital, try to find time to go out to dinner or a theater, or to engage in other social activities you both enjoy. Do not let the baby diminish the enjoyment you feel in each other's presence.

I know of husbands and wives who did not get along well together early in their marriage but who were united by the common bond of parenthood. The coming of babies gave them a cement of mutual interest and enabled them to curb their selfish impulses and to intensify their love for each other for the welfare of the family as a whole. Husbands and wives usually find greater pleasure in each other's company after a child is born. Now they have a source of unending mutual interest— the marvelous experience of watching their baby grow and develop new capabilities before their eyes.

I have also known of a few instances where a new baby was allowed to disrupt a marriage relationship which had seemed to be going smoothly. Some husbands and wives need constant reassurance of their mate's concern and interest in them. This is true in a small percentage of cases—but enough of them, unfortunately, to warrant a warning against allowing your infant to occupy so much of your attention that your spouse comes to think you are not as interested in him as you were before.

The "baby blues." Probably every mother must fight the urge to feel despondent after giving birth. There is often a certain amount of depression in the hospital just after the baby is born and then at home, when the new mother must begin to establish a strange new routine. In fact, this tendency to feel "low" is so common that there is a name for it—the "new baby blues."

You can deal with such a situation better if you realize that it is (a) normal and (b) caused, at least partially, by physical factors. You probably are aware of the effect that physiological changes can have upon your emotions and the way you look at life. For example, many women experience great emotional tension in the few days preceding menstruation. Some are tense, jittery, more inclined to see the "dark side" than at other times.

Perhaps you have noticed that problems of your own, which you generally can shrug off with a smile, may suddenly become so enormous before menstruation begins that you do not know how you can cope with them. Then you awaken one morning and the problems do not seem so difficult and overwhelming after all. What has happened, of course, is that your physical condition has had a pronounced effect upon your outlook. So it is during pregnancy. The extra activities of your glands, the increased secretion of hormones, the additional burdens placed upon your organs to accommodate the growing fetus —all these may affect your emotions. At the end of the pregnancy, the hormones of the endocrine system work to their highest capacity. After delivery, the system slows down rapidly. After every birth there is a period similar to the pre-menopause of later years.

In addition, there is a normal letdown that follows the ultimate achievement of something you have been anticipating for a long time. Many women will remember the nervous tension that built up just before marriage, and the inevitable letdown when the excitement was over and they were face to face with a strange new kind of life.

The "blues" that occur a few days after the baby is born generally result from a similar letdown. They also have a physical origin. At this time, your breasts may be beginning to fill up with milk and other changes are taking place as your body returns to normal. Do not be surprised if you feel the urge to weep for no particular reason.

Nor should you be surprised if you now suddenly notice a changed attitude toward your husband. You may feel that he is not as attentive as he might be, that he has been "having a good time" while you have gone through the agonies of childbirth, and that the arrangement which puts you in the hospital while he goes about his business is unfair for women generally. You may develop a sudden antipathy to other relatives, finding character flaws you had not been aware of before. Or you may become highly critical of the hospital staff. Although normally easygoing, you demand things which you really know are quite unreasonable to expect.

Many new mothers have a "good cry" or two in the hospital and report that they feel much more relaxed when it is over. You will feel less troubled by the "blues" if you realize that they will pass away.

You may also experience a sense of depression after you return home, when problems of caring for the baby present themselves. Here again, changes in your glandular system may be at least partially responsible. Some women feel depression most keenly when they realize that the need to care for their baby forces them to cancel their accustomed activities. They wonder if they will ever again be able to spend a relaxed afternoon shopping, visiting with friends, or engaging in other pleasures.

It will help your emotions if you can give yourself a few hours' "vacation" from the baby occasionally. You should not become a prisoner. Perhaps your relatives or friends will care for him during his nap, while you shop, visit friends, or engage in other social activities. Perhaps your husband will take charge for an evening while you go "out with the girls." Perhaps you can obtain a competent baby-sitter while you go out with your husband.

Don't allow yourself to develop a feeling of martyrdom. Learn to recognize the symptoms of self-pity—of feeling sorry for yourself, of comparing your responsibilities now with your freedom before the baby came, of measuring the way you seem to be chained down against the freedom from responsibility which your husband seems to have. It is true that you will have a more direct responsibility for your infant's well-being, but he also has the problem of supporting the new member of the family. Moreover, while your work will now be greater, so will your satisfactions.

Do not hesitate to consult your doctor if the feeling of depression persists for an unreasonable period of time, or if you consistently find yourself seeing faults in your husband or feeling incapable of handling your responsibilities of parenthood. Thanks to the advances of modern medicine, complications after birth can be treated as successfully as those during your pregnancy.

The art of maintaining a cheerful outlook is one you will find useful not only during your pregnancy, but throughout the rest of your life as well. You will have some trials, difficulties and disappointments in the future. I can say this with certainty because everyone does. Some of us have greater burdens than others, but I have never met anyone who could not ease his lot in life—and the lot of those around him—by looking upon the bright side of things. On the other hand, I have known those who experienced only the normal difficulties all of us must bear, but who gave them an air of catastrophe—all because of their depressing attitude.

Your serene outlook will actually help you do a better job as a mother. It is the calm, poised woman who takes the normal procedure of pregnancy in her stride. It is she who is able to feed her child from her breast. It is she who can care for him with an easy assurance which the child himself comes to sense and which, in turn, gives him the confidence to live his own full and happy life.

5

Terms Your Doctor May Use

Your doctor will strive to explain your progress in pregnancy and to instruct you in words which the average young mother-to-be can understand. Since it is important for your treatment that you understand clearly what he tells you, do not hesitate to ask that he explain any words or phrases which are unknown to you. Below are definitions of terms that obstetricians often use and with which patients may not be familiar.

Abdomen The front region of the body below the lower rib which contains most of the digestive organs. It is not correct to refer to this part as the stomach, as many persons do.

Abortion The expulsion of the fetus before it can live outside the body. Abortion is the technical term for miscarriage in the early stages of pregnancy. When involuntary, the abortion is referred to as spontaneous. When deliberate, it is a mortal sin for which absolution can be obtained only from a bishop.

Afterbirth The placenta and membrane which are expelled from the uterus after the baby is delivered.

Aftercare This term refers to the medical and nursing care of the mother after birth. It may also be called postnatal or postpartum care.

Anemia A blood condition, which can be detected by tests, in which there is an insufficient amount of hemoglobin or red blood cells.

Anesthesia   A medicine used to dull the sense of pain in the person to whom it is administered. A general anesthetic, such as gas or ether, puts the patient to sleep. Local anesthetics, injected beneath the skin or into the spinal canal, deaden specific areas of the body.

Bag of waters   Another term for the membrane which encloses the baby in the uterus. It is attached to the placenta and is filled with fluid.

Bladder   The organ which stores urine as it comes from the kidneys. The urine remains here until it is discharged from the body.

Blood pressure   The force exerted by the blood in the arteries. It is caused by the pumping of the heart and movement of blood in the body and can be measured accurately.

Breech baby   One born with either his feet or buttocks first. In the more usual method of birth, the head emerges from the mother's body first.

Bunting   An outer wrap for a baby. It usually is a hood to which a blanket is attached.

Catheterization   The process by which a tube is passed through the urethra into the bladder in order to extract urine.

Cervix   The lower, narrow end of the womb. It opens into the vagina.

Circumcision   The operation by which the foreskin of the penis is removed.

Caesarean section   A birth in which the baby is removed from the uterus by means of an abdominal operation.

Clitoris   A part of the vulva, located just above the opening.

Colostrum   A watery fluid which may begin to seep from the mother's nipples around the fourth month of pregnancy. Colostrum can nourish a newborn baby until the mother's real milk begins to form a few days after birth.

Conception The union of the male sperm and female egg to form a new human life.

Confinement The period during which labor and birth occur.

Convalescence In this instance, the period of recovery after childbirth. The term can also refer to the recovery period after any operation or illness.

Delivery Birth of the baby.

Ducts Passages through which the eggs travel from the ovaries and the sperm travel from the testicles.

Dysmenorrhea Painful menstruation.

Dyspareunia Painful sexual intercourse.

Embryo The fertilized egg during the first three months of development.

Endometrial biopsy An excision or scraping which the physician takes from the lining of the uterus.

Episiotomy A small cut which the physician makes at the opening of the mother's vagina at birth to enable the baby to be born without tearing her skin.

Estrogen The hormones responsible for the development of feminine characteristics.

Fallopian tubes The passages in which the egg moves from the ovary to the womb.

Fertilization The penetration by the male sperm into the nucleus of the female egg in the act of conception.

Fetus The unborn child after about the third month of its development.

Follicle The area in the ovary in which the egg matures until it is discharged in ovulation.

Foreskin The skin which covers the head of the penis. This is the part which is removed in circumcision.

Fontanelle The spot on the top center of the baby's head which is soft at birth. The bones of the skull require several months to grow together.

Forceps   An instrument sometimes used to lift the baby's head out of the vagina during birth.

Glans   The sensitive head of the clitoris or penis.

Hemoglobin   The red matter in the blood which transports oxygen.

Hormone   A secretion of any of the ductless glands. Hormones regulate many different activities of the body.

Involution   The process by which the uterus regains its former size after birth.

Kidneys   Two organs of the body located on each side of the backbone near the waistline. Kidneys are responsible for the formation of urine.

Labor   The final stage of pregnancy immediately preceding the birth of the baby. Labor serves to enlarge the uterus and cervix to enable the baby to pass through.

Leucorrhea   A whitish discharge from the vagina which results from infection.

Lightening   Movement of the baby lower into the abdomen in the last stages of pregnancy.

Lochia   A discharge of blood and tissue from the uterus after the baby is born.

Maternity care   The term used to describe the general services of the obstetrician—the care of an expectant mother before, during and after the baby's birth.

Meatus   An opening, such as that of the cervix into the vagina.

Menopause   The period of change a woman experiences when her ovaries cease to produce eggs, thus making her incapable of conceiving and of menstruating.

Menses   The regular process in which the uterine lining is disposed of if the egg has not been fertilized.

Minerals   Elements such as iron, calcium and phosphorus, which are present in foods and in body cells.

Miscarriage A delivery during the early stages of pregnancy, before the baby has developed so that it could survive outside the womb.

"Mittelschmerz" The twinge of "middle pain" some women feel at ovulation. When they have this pain, they know that the egg has been discharged from the ovary.

Morning sickness A sense of nausea or discomfort felt in the morning, which may occur during the early part of pregnancy.

Mucous membrane A thin membrane lining which exists in the mouth, nose, vagina and inside the digestive tract.

Mucous The material which keeps the mucous membrane moist. It is secreted by glands.

Nausea A sense of discomfort in the stomach associated with a desire to vomit.

Obstetrician A doctor who cares for women before, during and immediately after they deliver a baby.

Ovaries Two organs which prepare the eggs in the female.

Oviducts The Fallopian tubes, passageway for the eggs moving from the ovaries to the uterus.

Ovulation The process by which the egg is discharged from the ovary.

Ovum The female egg, or sex cell.

Penis The male organ of generation.

Pelvic examination The doctor's examination of the womb and ovaries.

Pelvic measurements A measurement by the doctor to determine the size of the birth canal.

Pelvic organs The organs which lie between the pelvic bones—uterus, vagina, ovaries, Fallopian tubes, bladder and rectum.

Pelvis The circle of bone at the base of the trunk. The leg bones are attached to it.

Placenta　The organ attached to the lining of the uterus. The unborn child gets nourishment from it through the umbilical cord.

Postpartum examination　An examination made after birth by the doctor to make certain that the pelvic organs are again normal.

Pregnancy　The period from the time of conception until birth or miscarriage.

Rubin Test　A method widely used by doctors to examine a woman's Fallopian tubes to determine if there is any blockage there.

Prenatal care　Medical supervision by a doctor during pregnancy.

Pubic bone　The front bone of the pelvis.

Rectum　The lower end of the bowel.

Rhythm method　A means of avoiding conception by making use of the sterile periods in the female menstrual cycle.

Scrotum　The bag in which the testes are normally found.

Semen　The fluid secreted by the male in the sexual act.

Seminal pool　The concentration of deposited semen in the upper vagina, usually in contact with the cervix.

"Show"　A small quantity of blood and mucous which is discharged early in labor.

Smegma　A secretion which is generally concentrated in the foreskin of the penis and the folds of the clitoris.

Sperm　A term used to denote a single spermatozoön as well as a collection of sperm cells.

Sphincter muscle　A muscle at the base of the bowel. It controls the evacuation of the bowel.

Stethoscope　The instrument the doctor uses to detect heartbeats, breath sounds and other noises from inside the body.

Tampon　A preparation of cotton which is inserted into the vagina. It may absorb menstrual flow, apply medicine to the vagina or cervix, or may be used with a test tape to determine the time of ovulation.

Testes (testicles) Two male organs which produce sperm.

Testosterone Main male hormone.

Trichomonas An infection of the vagina.

Umbilical cord The cord which connects the baby's abdomen with the placenta. It carries the baby's blood to and from the placenta.

Urethra The passage through which urine passes from the bladder to the outside of the body.

Uterus The organ, also called the womb, in which the baby develops until birth.

Vagina The canal which extends from the uterus to the outside of the body, through which the baby passes at birth.

Vestibule Erectile tissue around the opening of the vagina.

Vernix A creamy substance which covers the baby's skin at birth.

Vulva A term used to describe a woman's external genitals.

Womb Also called the uterus. The organ in which a fertilized egg settles and develops until birth.

6

Your Guide to Weight Control

Your doctor will want you to watch your weight carefully during pregnancy. The expectant mother who gains too much weight may tire easily and become excessively uncomfortable as the date of birth approaches. It is usually recommended that she begin to check her food consumption as soon as the doctor verifies that she is pregnant.

Millions of words have been written on the subject, but weight control remains a simple question of arithmetic. Your body needs so many calories each day to give you the energy to live. How many calories you need depends upon many factors: your height, your type of body build, the amount of activities in which you engage and your metabolic rate—the measurement of your body's efficiency in converting food into energy.

A typical pregnant woman requires about 2,500 calories per day. If she regularly eats more than she needs, the excess will be stored in her body as fat. If she consumes less than she needs, the balance required to keep her body functioning will be taken from what is stored in her body.

When you gain weight, you have eaten more calories than your body needs for its normal functioning. To lose weight, you must take in fewer calories than you need so that the rest can be supplied from your fat. It is important, therefore, to know the caloric values of the various foods you eat. The guide below will enable you to control your intake wisely.

Never embark upon any diet during pregnancy without first consulting your doctor. An expectant mother who starts a fad diet without her doctor's knowledge and approval may be creating serious difficulties for herself.

Your doctor may provide you with a list of typical meals you can eat to keep your weight within reasonable limits. He will weigh you on each of your visits and let you know whether you are making the progress expected of you. The following guide lists individual items followed by the caloric content.

BEVERAGES (Nonalcoholic—All 8-oz. portions.)
Buttermilk   87
Chocolate-flavored milk   185
Cider   120
Club soda (carbonated water)   0
Condensed milk, sweetened and undiluted   980
Cocoa made with milk   235
Cocoa made with milk and water   140
Coffee, black, unsweetened   0
Coffee with 1 tablespoon light cream, 1 teaspoon sugar   50
Coffee with 1 tablespoon heavy cream, 1 teaspoon sugar   65
Coffee with scant teaspoon of sugar   16
Evaporated milk, undiluted   345
Ginger ale   80
Grapefruit juice, sweetened   130
Grapefruit juice, unsweetened   90
Grapefruit-orange juice blend, sweetened   130
Grapefruit-orange juice blend, unsweetened   100
Lemonade, sweet   100
Milk, whole   166
Milk shake   280
Skim milk   87
Soft drinks (except noncaloric kinds)   104

BEVERAGES (Continued)

Tea with lemon   5
Tea with ¼ cup milk   40
Tomato juice   50
Sauerkraut juice, ½ cup   3

BREADS (Calories per slice of approximately ½ inch unless otherwise noted.)

Boston brown bread, per oz.   60
Cracked wheat   60
Date and nut, small slice   80
French or Vienna, 1oz.   75
Gluten bread   65
Graham   65
Italian bread, 1 oz.   75
Pumpernickel   95
Raisin   65
Rye, American   60
White   65
Whole wheat   60
Melba toast, slice 4 in. square   40

BUTTER, MARGARINE AND LARD

Butter and margarine, 1 tablespoon   100
Butter and margarine, 1 pat or square, 64 to pound   50
Lard, 1 tablespoon   125

CAKES

Angel food, 2-in. sector of 8-in. cake   110
Cheese cake, 2-in. wedge   200
Cream puff (medium size)   250
Devil's food, 2-in. sector of 8-in. cake   120
Doughnut, 1 small   135
Fruit cake, 1-oz. piece 2 x 2 x ½ in.   105
Gingerbread, 2-in. square, 1 in. thick   110
Jelly roll, ½-in. slice 3¼ in. diameter   180
Layer cake, chocolate, 2-in. sector of 8-in. cake   320
Pound cake, 1-oz. slice   130
Spice cake, 2-in. cube   190

CAKES (Continued)
Sponge cake, 2-in. sector of 8-in. cake   115
Cupcake, large   160

CANDIES (All individual pieces unless otherwise indicated.)
Butterscotch   20
Caramel   40
Chocolate cream, small   55
Chocolate mint, 1½-in. diameter   30
Fudge, 1 medium-size square   50
Gumdrop, ½-in. diameter   30
Hard candy, 1 oz.   110
Jelly bean, 1 large   17
Lollipop, average   75
Marshmallow, 1   20
Milk chocolate, plain, 1 oz.   143
Milk chocolate, with almonds, 1 oz.   150
Mint, cream   20
Peanut brittle, 1 oz.   125

CEREALS (All ¼-cup [2 oz.] portions unless otherwise indicated.)
Barley, cooked   40
Barley, pearled, dry   85
Bran flakes   30
Bran, raisin   38
Corn flakes   24
Cracked wheat, cooked   41
Cream of wheat, cooked   41
Farina, cooked   27
Grapenuts   102
Maltex, cooked   42
Oatmeal or rolled oats, cooked   42
Oat cereal, ready-to-eat   25
Puffed rice   17
Puffed wheat   12
Rice, brown, raw   180
Rice, white, raw   170

CEREALS (Continued)
Rice flakes 26
Rolled wheat, cooked 42
Shredded wheat (large biscuit) 105
Shredded wheat (small biscuit) 80

CHEESE (All 1-oz. portions unless otherwise indicated.)
Blue cheese 105
Blue mold 105
Brick 100
Camembert 110
Cheddar (1-in. cube) 80
Cottage cheese 27
Cream cheese (1 tablespoon) 75
Gruyère 105
Liederkranz (1 tablespoon) 45
Limburger 95
Parmesan 110
Parmesan, grated (1 tablespoon) 20
Pimento (1-in. cube) 75
Pineapple (1-in. cube) 90
Roquefort (1-in. cube) 40
Swiss 105
Cheese foods (processed cheddar) 90

COOKIES (Calories per piece)
Assorted, average 45
Brownies, average 50
Chocolate wafer 35
Fig bar, large 85
Gingersnap, 1¾-in. diameter 20
Icebox, ⅓ oz. 45
Macaroon, coconut, 1-in. diameter 45

CRACKERS (Calories per piece)
Butter cracker, round 15
Cheese bit 7
Graham, chocolate-covered, large 70

CRACKERS (Continued)
Oatmeal, round   25
Oyster   4
Pretzel, large   50
Soda, 2½-in. square   23

CREAM
Light, 1 tablespoon   30
Heavy or whipping, 1 tablespoon   50
Whipped cream, 1 tablespoon   35

DESSERTS
Gelatin
   Plain, unsweetened, dry, 1 tablespoon   35
   Sweetened dessert powder, 3-oz. pkg., ½ cup   32
Ice Cream (*all flavors, plain, commercial*)
   Scoop, 2½-in. diameter   105
   Ice cream soda (average)   300
   Ice cream sundae (average, with syrup, chopped nuts)   350
   Ices: Fruit juice, sugar, water, ½ cup   115
Puddings (*all 4-oz. portions*)
   Bread, rich   200
   Chocolate cornstarch   160
   Cornstarch   140
   Custard cup, baked or boiled   115
   Fig   400
   Plum   345
   Rice, creamy   185
   Tapioca, creamy   130
   Vanilla, cornstarch   140
Sherbet
   ¼ pint   120
   Small scoop   60

EGGS (Calories are for one hen's egg.)
Deviled egg   90
Hard-boiled egg   77
White of egg   15

E G G S (Continued)
Yolk of egg   62
Omelet   105
Poached egg   77
Raw egg   77
Scrambled egg   105

F I S H (All servings of 4 oz. unless otherwise indicated.)
Bass, sea   105
Bluefish, baked   195
Bluefish, fried   280
Clams, Cherrystone, 6 medium   65
Clams, Little Neck, 6 small   55
Clams, long, soft shell, 6 large (½ cup)   100
Clam juice, canned, ½ cup   14
Cod, dried   150
Cod, fresh   95
Codfish balls (per ball, 2-in. diameter)   100
Codfish, creamed   150
Flounder, fillet   75
Haddock, fillet   215
Halibut, steak, 4 oz.   225
Herring, Atlantic   215
Herring, lake   160
Herring, Pacific   105
Herring, smoked kippered   240
Kingfish   100
Lobster, boiled, (edible 4 ozs.)   90
Mackerel, fresh   165
Mackerel, salt   340
Oysters on half-shell, 6 with sauce   100
Oysters, fried, 6 small   250
Porgy   150
Red snapper   100
Salmon, canned Chinook or King, 3 ozs.   175
Salmon, canned pink or Humpback Chum, 3 ozs.   120
Salmon, canned Choho, silver, Sockeye or red, 3 ozs.   142

FISH (Continued)
Salmon, fresh Pacific, broiled or baked, 1 steak 4 x 3 x ½   205
Sardines, Atlantic type, canned in oil, solids and liquids, 3 ozs.   290
Sardines, Pacific type, canned, solids and liquid   170
Scallops   90
Shad   190
Shrimp, canned, 8 medium   75
Shrimp, fresh, 8 medium   60
Swordfish, broiled, 1 steak 3 x 3 x ½ in.   225
Trout, brook, broiled   130
Tuna, canned (solids only)   230
Tuna, canned (solids and liquids)   335
Weakfish, steamed   115
Whitefish, steamed   115

FLOUR (Calories are for 1 cup.)
Buckwheat   340
Cake   385
Corn   405
Pastry   385
Potato   470
Rice   550
Rye   285
Wheat, general-purpose white   400
Wheat, self-rising   385
Whole wheat   400

FRUITS
Apple, raw, 1 medium, 2½-in. diameter   75
Applesauce, canned, sweetened, ½ cup   90
Apple juice, 8 oz.   120
Apricots, canned, syrup pack, 4 medium halves, 2 tablespoons syrup   95
Apricots, dried, small halves, each   10
Apricots, raw, 1 large   20
Banana, 1, 6 in.   90
Blueberries, canned, syrup pack, 1 cup with liquid   245

FRUITS (Continued)

Blueberries, fresh, 1 cup   85

Cherries, canned, sour, pitted, 1 cup with liquid   120

Cherries, sour, raw, whole, 1 cup   65

Cherries, sweet, 1 raw, large   4

Cherries, maraschino, 1   5

Coconut, shredded, 1 cup   345

Cranberries, raw, 1 cup   55

Dates, fresh or dried, 1 oz.   75

Fruit cocktail, canned, solids and liquid, ½ cup   90

Gooseberries, canned in syrup, ½ cup   90

Gooseberries, raw, 1 cup   60

Grapefruit, canned, sweetened, solids and liquid, ½ cup   90

Grapefruit, one half of fruit, 4-in. diameter   50

Grapefruit sections, 1 cup   75

Grapes, type with slip skin (Concord, Delaware, Niagara, etc.), 1 bunch, 3½ ozs.   55

Grapes, type with adherent skin (Malaga, Muscat, Tokay, Thompson seedless, etc.), each grape ¾ in. in diameter   2½

Honeydew melon, 1 wedge (2 x 7 in.)   50

Lemon, 1 medium (3 oz.)   20

Loganberries, raw, 1 cup   90

Muskmelon (cantaloupe), one half of 5-inch melon   40

Olive, green, "mammoth size," 1   7

Olive, ripe, Mission, 1   10

Olives, other varieties (Ascalano, Manzanilla, Sevilano), 1   7

Orange, raw, 1 medium, 3 in. in diameter   70

Orange sections, 1 cup   85

Peach, dried, small half   25

Peach, fresh, 1 medium (2 x 2½)   45

Peaches, canned with syrup (2 medium halves, 2 tablespoons syrup)   175

Pear, dried, one half   60

Pear, fresh, 1 medium (3 x 2½ in.)   95

Pears, canned with syrup (2 med. halves, 2 tablespoons syrup)   80

Pineapple, canned with syrup, 1 large slice, 2 tablespoons juice   95

Pineapple, canned with syrup, 1 cup crushed   205

FRUITS (Continued)

Pineapple, fresh, 1 slice 3½-in. diameter   45
Plum, fresh, 1, 2-in. diameter   30
Plums, canned, syrup pack, 2 plums and juice   80
Plums, Italian prune type, canned with syrup, 2 prunes without
   pits, 2 tablespoons juice   70
Prune, fresh, 1 large   24
Prune, fresh, 1 small   14
Raspberries, black, fresh, 1 cup   50
Raspberries, black, canned with syrup, ½ cup   125
Strawberries, fresh, whole, 1 cup   55
Strawberries, canned with syrup, ½ cup   115
Tangerine, fresh, 1 medium (2½-in. diameter)   35
Watermelon, 1 slice 2 in. wide by 10 in. long   115

MEATS AND POULTRY

Bacon, medium-fat, crisp-fried, drained, 1 slice   45
Bacon, Canadian, 1 slice, 2½ x ⁹⁄₁₆   115
Beef, canned
   Corned beef, 3 ozs.   245
   Corned-beef hash, 3 ozs.   120
   Roast beef, 3 ozs.   190
Beef roasts (*medium-fat, average servings 4 ozs., edible portion*)
   Loin roasts   390
   Pot roast (round)   230
   Rib roast   290
Beef steaks (*medium-fat, average serving 4 ozs., edible portion*)
   Club   220
   Porterhouse   330
   Rib (T-bone)   320
   Round   230
   Rump   390
   Sirloin   275
   Swiss   345
Beef broth, 1 cup   120
Beef liver, fried, 4 ozs.   220
Bologna, 1 oz., slice ⅛ in. thick, 4½-in. diameter   65

MEATS AND POULTRY (Continued)

Bouillon, 1 cup   10
Bouillon cubes, 1 cube   2
Brains, all kinds, fresh, 3 ozs.   105
Chicken
    Broiler, half (8 ozs. without bone)   330
    Fryer, average size, breast   210
    Fryer, average size, leg   160
    Giblets, ⅓ cup   160
    Gizzard, 1 average   50
    Liver, 1 medium   50
    Roaster, ½ breast   200
    Roaster, 3 average slices   175
    Roaster, average thigh or leg   180
Frankfurter, 5½ in.   120
Hamburger, average 2-oz. patty   210
Hamburger, lean ground round, 2 oz.   140
Heart (*all 3-oz. portions*)
    Beef, lean with visible fat   190
    Chicken   135
    Lamb or mutton   130
    Pork   100
    Veal   160
Kidneys (*all 3-oz. portions*)
    Beef   120
    Pork   100
    Sheep   90
    Veal   110
Lamb (*all 3-oz. portions*)
    Rib chop   350
    Shoulder chop   290
    Leg roast without bone   230
    Shoulder roast without bone   295
    Stew meat (breast)   325
Liver
    Beef, fried, 3 ozs.   175
    Calf or veal, 3 ozs.   160
    Chicken, 1 medium   50

MEATS AND POULTRY (Continued)

Liver (*Continued*)
    Lamb or sheep, 3 ozs.   150
    Pork, 3 ozs.   150
    Liver, 2 ozs.   150
Luncheon meat, spiced, 1 oz. (slice ⅛ x 4 x 3½)   80
Meatball, 1, 1½-in. diameter   160
Meat loaf, ½ cup   160
Meat pie, ½ cup, with biscuit   400
Meat stock, 1 cup   25
Mutton
    Chop, lean, cooked   135
    Leg, roast, 3 ozs.   230
Pork
    Boiled ham, 1 slice, ⅛ in. thick   45
    Smoked ham, 1 slice, 4½ x 4⅜   385
    Boston butt, 1 slice, 4½ x 3½ x ⅓   350
    Chops, 1 medium, ½ in. thick   350
    Ham, lean, 1 slice, 5 x 5 x ¼   350
    Loin, roasted, 1 piece 3¼ x 3 x ⅓   350
    Picnic ham, 1 slice, 4½ x 3½ x ⅓   350
    Salt pork, 1-in. cube   135
Rabbit
    Domesticated, 3½ ozs.   175
    Wild, 3½ ozs.   130
Link sausage, Liverwurst, 1 oz. (1 slice, ¼ in. thick, 3-in. diameter)
    75
Salami, 1 oz. (1 slice ¹⁄₁₆ in. thick, 3-in. diameter)   55
Sausage patty (country sausage) 1 patty ½ in. thick, 2-in. diameter
    270
Sausage, summer, 1 oz.   125
Sausage, Vienna, approx. 5   245
Spareribs, 5 pcs. 4 x 1 in.   415
Tripe, beef, cooked, 4 ozs.   105
Tripe, beef, canned, 4 ozs.   170
Turkey
    Medium fat, raw, 4 ozs.   300
    Roasted, 2 ozs. (slice 4 x 2½ x ¼)   145

MEATS AND POULTRY (Continued)

Turkey (*Continued*)

    Giblets, ⅓ cup   160

Veal

    Chops, 1 average medium-fat   180

    Cutlet, roasted, 1 average   180

    Roast, 2 ozs. (slice 4 x 2½ x ½)   150

    Roasted, 1 average, fat removed   120

    Stew meat, 3 ozs. without bone   250

    Veal stew with vegetables, 1 cup   180

MISCELLANEOUS FOODS (Calories are for 1 tablespoon unless otherwise indicated.)

Catsup, tomato   17

Chives, fresh, ½ cup   25

Cooking oils (corn, cottonseed, olive, peanut, soy)   125

Cornstarch   30

Corn syrup   55

Curry sauce   25

Gravy, pan   20

Gravy with milk   60

Gravy with water   20

Jams   55

Jellies   50

Maple syrup   50

Marmalade   55

Mineral oil   0

Molasses, Blackstrap   43

Molasses, light   50

Molasses, medium-dark   46

Mustard, yellow, 1 teaspoon   5

Oils, salad or cooking (corn, cottonseed, olive, peanut, soy, etc.)   125

Pepper   Almost 0

Relish   30

Salad oils (olive, corn, peanut, soy, etc.)   125

Salt   Almost 0

MISCELLANEOUS FOODS (Continued)
Vinegar   Almost 0
White sauce, medium   25
Yeast, Brewer's, dry   22

MUFFINS (Calories per individual piece.)
Blueberry, 2-in. diameter   50
Bran, 2¼-in. diameter   90
Corn, 2¾-in. diameter   105
English, 2-oz. size   160
Plain, 2¾-in. diameter   130

NUTS (Calories per nut unless otherwise indicated.)
Almond, salted   8
Black walnut   40
Brazil nut   28
Cashews, roasted, 1 oz.   165
Chestnut, fresh   10
Filbert   8
Hazelnut   7
Hickory nut   8
Peanut, Virginia, whole   9
Peanuts, Spanish, 1 tablespoon   45
Pistachio nuts, 1 oz. kernels   180
Walnut, English, large   30

PANCAKES AND PASTA
Buckwheat griddlecake, 1, 4½-in. diameter, plain   95
Buckwheat griddlecake, 1, 4½-in. diameter with 1 pat butter and
   1 tablespoon maple syrup   195
Wheatcake, 1, 4-in. diameter   80
Wheatcake, 1, with butter and syrup   180
Waffles, 1 segment, dry   95
Waffles, 1 segment, with 1 pat butter and 1 tablespoon syrup   195
Macaroni, cooked, 1 cup elbow type or 1-in. pieces   210
Macaroni and cheese, baked, ½ cup   230
Macaroni and tomato sauce, ½ cup   150

PANCAKES AND PASTA (Continued)
Noodles, egg, cooked, 1 cup   110
Noodles, cooked, 1 pound   300
Noodles, dry, 1 cup   280
Spaghetti, cooked, 1 cup   220

PIES (All with double crust. Calories given are for a normal serving—one sixth of a pie 9 in. in diameter.)
Apple   385
Blueberry   340
Cherry   395
Coconut Custard   310
Cranberry   405
Custard   310
Lemon meringue   350
Mince   395
Peach   330
Pumpkin   310
Raisin   320
Rhubarb   310

ROLLS AND LIGHT PASTRIES (Calories per piece unless otherwise indicated.)
Cinnamon bun   100
Coffee cake, 2 ozs.   140
Hard roll, large   105
Jelly roll, ½-in. slice 3¼-in. diameter   180
Soft roll, plain, 2 ozs.   160
Popover   100
Sweet roll, 2 ozs.   180
Whole wheat roll, medium   95
Spice cake, 2-in. cube   190

SALADS (All ½ cup unless otherwise indicated.)
Asparagus, 6 spears with mayonnaise   110
Chicken, with mayonnaise   150
Coleslaw, with boiled dressing   40
Coleslaw, with cream and vinegar dressing   45

SALADS (Continued)

Cottage cheese on pineapple slice   80
Crabmeat, with mayonnaise   150
Egg salad (lettuce with 1 egg and 1 tablespoon mayonnaise)   175
Fruit, with mayonnaise   150
Lettuce, one quarter head with French dressing   75
Lobster, with mayonnaise   150
Potato salad   200
Shrimp with mayonnaise   150
Tomatoes, cucumber, lettuce, French dressing   100
Tuna   180
Vegetables, mixed with French dressing   90
Waldorf   180

SALAD DRESSINGS (All 1-tablespoon portions.)

Commercial, plain (mayonnaise type)   60
French   60
Home-cooked, boiled   28
Mayonnaise   92
Roquefort   110
Russian   65
Tartar sauce   100
Thousand Island   50
Tomato catsup with lemon juice   15

SANDWICHES (All include approximately one ounce of the filler indicated, either a pat of butter or ½ tablespoon of mayonnaise, and two standard slices of white or brown bread unless otherwise indicated. Calorie values of lettuce, pickles, relish, catsup and mustard added to sandwiches usually are almost negligible.)

Bacon and tomato   260
Beef, cold slices   265
Boiled ham (thin slice)   220
Bologna   240
Cheese, cheddar (processed, ⅛-inch slice)   235
Chicken, cold   275
Chicken, hot, with gravy   300
Chicken salad   225

SANDWICHES (Continued)
Club (three-decker)   375
Cold cuts   275
Corned beef   260
Cream cheese (soft cream spreads)   200
Deviled ham   250
Egg salad   225
Frankfurter and roll   215
Ham and cheese (thin slice boiled ham, cheese)   285
Ham, baked (⅛-inch slice)   300
Ham, boiled (thin slice)   220
Hamburger and bun   225
Jelly, plain   225
Lettuce and tomato   190
Liverwurst   275
Peanut butter   225
Peanut butter and jelly   275
Roast beef, cold   265
Roast beef, hot, with gravy   300
Salami   295
Sardine   250
Swiss cheese   260
Tongue (2 slices)   275
Tuna (shredded)   265
Turkey, cold   275
Turkey, hot, with gravy   300

SOUPS (All 1-cup portions.)
Asparagus, cream   200
Bean   190
Beef   100
Bouillon and broth   10
Celery, cream   200
Chicken   75
Chicken noodle   140
Clam chowder   85
Consommé   10

S O U P S (Continued)
Corn, cream   300
Lentil   550
Mushroom, cream   200
Noodle   120
Onion   105
Oxtail   190
Pea   140
Rice   120
Spinach, cream   200
Tomato, cream   200
Tomato, plain   90
Vegetable   85

S U G A R S (All 1-tablespoon portions.)
Brown, light or dark   50
Cane or beet, granulated   48
Powdered (confectioner's)   31

S Y R U P S (All 1-tablespoon portions.)
Chocolate   42
Corn   60
Maple   50
Molasses, light   50
Sorghum   55

V E G E T A B L E S
Asparagus (1 5-in. stalk)   2
Avocado, half of 1 medium   275
Beans
   Baked, canned, pork and molasses, ½ cup   160
   Baked, canned, pork and tomato sauce, ½ cup   145
   Green beans (snap or wax), canned, 1 cup (with liquids, 16 calories)   43
   Kidney beans, canned or cooked, ½ cup   115
   Lima beans, canned, ½ cup (with liquids, 15 calories)   90
   Cooked, ½ cup   75
   Dry mature seeds, 1 cup   610

VEGETABLES (Continued)

Beans (*Continued*)

  Navy, pea beans, dry, ½ cup   320

Broccoli, 1 medium stalk   25

Brussels sprout, 1 medium-size   8

Cabbage, cooked, 1 cup   40

Cabbage, red or white, raw, 1 cup finely shredded   25

Carrot, raw, 6 in.   23

Carrots, 1 cup diced, cooked   45

Cauliflower, cooked, 1 cup   30

Celery, 1 stalk, 8 in. long   8

Chard, leaves and stalks, cooked, 1 cup   30

Chicory (curly endive), 3 leaves   2

Corn, solids and liquid, 1 cup   170

Corn, 1 ear, 5 in. long   85

Cucumber, 1, 7½ in.   25

Cucumber pickle, 1, 4 in. long   18

Dandelion greens, 1 cup cooked   75

Endive, raw, 1 leaf   1

Escarole, 1 leaf   3

Leek, 1, 5 in. long   15

Lentils, 1 tablespoon dry   50

Lettuce, 1 small leaf   2

Mustard greens, cooked, 1 cup   30

Onion, green, young, 1   4

Onion, mature, raw, 1, 2½-in. diameter   50

Peas, canned, solids and liquid, 1 cup   170

Peas, green, medium age, 1 cup   120

Peas, split (dry, mature seeds), ¼ cup   175

Pepper, green, 1 medium   20

Pepper, red, 1 medium   30

Pickles

  Dill, 1 large, 4 in. long   15

  Mustard pickles, 1 tablespoon   25

  Sour, 1 large, 4 in. long   15

  Sweet, 2 pickles, 2 in. long   22

VEGETABLES (Continued)

Potatoes (white)

Baked, 1, 2½-in. diameter   100

Boiled, 1, 2½-in. diameter or 1 cup diced   100

Dehydrated, 1 oz.   315

French fried, 8 pcs. 2 x ½ x ½   160

Fried raw (pan fried) ¼ cup   240

Hash brown, ½ cup   235

Mashed, with milk and butter added, ½ cup   120

Potato chips, 1 piece   8

Potato flour, 1 cup   470

Potatoes (sweet)

Baked, 1, 4 ozs. (5 x 2 in.)   185

Boiled, 1 (5 x 2½ in.)   250

Candied, 1 small (3½ x 2¼ in.)   315

Canned, 1 cup   235

Pumpkin, 1 cup   70

Radish, 1 small   1

Red cabbage, cooked, 1 cup   40

Red kidney beans, canned or cooked, ½ cup   115

Romaine, 1 leaf   2

Sauerkraut, solids and liquids, 1 cup   37

Soybeans, dried, mature, ½ cup   350

Soybeans, fresh, shelled, 1 cup   150

Spinach, canned, solids and liquid, or drained ½ cup   23

Spinach, fresh leaves, 1 cup   10

Squash, summer, cooked, 1 cup   35

Squash, winter, cooked, 1 cup   100

Succotash, canned or cooked, ½ cup   130

Tomato, raw, 1 medium (2 x 2½ in.)   30

Tomatoes, canned or cooked, ½ cup   23

Turnips, raw, ½ cup diced   22

Turnip greens, boiled, ½ cup   22

Water cress, raw, 1 cup   10

7

What Should You Name Your Baby?

Church law states that you should give your child a suitable name by which he will be addressed when he becomes a Christian at the time of his Baptism. This Christian name might be that of a saint, or one which recalls some great event in Biblical history. Unless he is given a Christian name, the pastor is directed to "add to the name given by the parents, the name of some saint and enter both in the Baptismal record."

As a practical matter, it would be wise to decide upon a name before the baby is born. You will be asked to provide a name for the hospital and Health Department records within a few days after birth.

Four points to help you make a good selection. There are thousands of Christian names to choose from, but not all are suitable for modern times and many might be inappropriate in your case. To help you make a satisfactory choice, the following principles might be kept in mind:

1. The name should be distinctly masculine or distinctly feminine. For example, Vivian is usually regarded as a girl's name and has proved a source of embarrassment when given to boys.

2. Select a name appropriate for your surname. For instance, a first name ending with "s" or "th" usually does not go well with a last name beginning the same way. A short first name often goes well with a long last name, and a long first name often best suits a short surname.

3. Consider whether your child's initials will spell something unpleasant. Mr. and Mrs. Tyler named their boy Robert Anthony. His playmates nicknamed him "Rat."

4. Consider the difficulties of a person with a common name which is difficult to spell. Parents sometimes choose a variation of a common name—the name Jonne, for instance, instead of John. A boy with such a name will go through life striving to correct everyone who spells his name in the usual way.

A selected list of names. Below is a careful compilation of appropriate boys' and girls' names for modern times. Also given is the source of the name, its original meaning, and the feast date of the saint from whom the name is derived. While this is only a partial list, an effort was made to include all names which seem appropriate for modern life. You may find a more complete section in a dictionary of saints.

BOYS' NAMES

AARON (Hebrew) *High mountain*, Oct. 9
ABEL (Hebrew) *Breath*, Jan. 2
ABELARD *a form of Abel*, Jan. 2
ABRAHAM (Hebrew) *Father of multitudes*, Oct. 9
ACHILLES (Greek) *One without lips*, Nov. 7
ADAM (Hebrew) *Man of the earth*, Dec. 24
ADDISON *a form of Adam*, Dec. 24
ADOLF *a form of Adolph*, Feb. 11

ADOLPH (German) *Noble wolf*, Feb. 11

ADRAM (Latin) *From Adria, Italy*, Jan. 9

ALAN (Celtic) *Comely or fair*, Oct. 26

ALBAN (Latin) *White*, June 21

ALBERT (German) *Noble and brilliant*, Nov. 15

ALBIAN (Celtic) *White cliff*, June 10

ALEXANDER (Greek) *Helper of mankind*, Mar. 18

ALEXIS (Greek) *Servant of men*, July 17

ALFONSO *a form of Alphonsus*, Aug. 2

ALGER (Anglo-Saxon) *Noble spearman*, Apr. 11

ALLAN *a form of Alan*, Oct. 26

ALLEN *a form of Alan*, Oct. 26

ALLISTER *a form of Alexander*, Mar. 18

ALPHONSO *a form of Alphonsus*, Aug. 2

ALPHONSUS (German) *Eager for battle*, Aug. 2

ALVIN (German) *Beloved by all*, Dec. 27

AMBROSE (Greek) *Immortal*, July 19

AMOS (Hebrew) *A burden*, Mar. 31

ANASTASIUS (Greek) *One who shall rise again*, Dec. 19

ANATOL *a form of Anatole*, June 3

ANATOLE (Greek) *From the East*, June 3

ANDERS *a form of Andrew*, Nov. 20

ANDERSON *a form of Andrew*, Nov. 20

ANDRE (Greek) *Manly*, Nov. 20

ANGELO *a form of Angelus*, Sept. 20

ANGELUS (Greek) *An angel*, Sept. 10

ANTHONY *a form of Antony*, Jan. 17

ANTON *a form of Antony*, Jan. 17

ANTONIO *a form of Antony*, Jan. 17

ANTONY (Latin) *Beyond praise*, Jan. 17

ARAM *a form of Abraham*, Oct. 9

ARCHIBALD (German) *Holy prince*, Apr. 20

ARNOLD (German) *Mighty as the eagle*, July 8

ATHANASIUS (Greek) *Immortal*, May 2

AUGUSTINE (Latin) *Sacred or sublime*, May 26

AUSTIN *a form of Augustine*, May 26

BARNABAS (Hebrew) *Son of prophecy*, June 11
BARNABY *a form of Barnabas*, June 11
BARNARD (German) *Firm bear*, Jan. 23
BARNEY *a form of Bernard*, Aug. 20
BARRY (Gaelic) *A form of Finbar, White head*, Sept. 25
BARTHOLOMEW (Hebrew) *Son of the furrows*, Aug. 24
BARTLEY *a form of Bartholomew*, Aug. 24
BARTON *a form of Bartholomew*, Aug. 24
BARTRAM *a form of Bertrand*, Sept. 6
BASIL (Greek) *Kingly*, June 14
BEDE (German) *Prayer*, May 27
BENEDICT (Latin) *Blessed*, Mar. 21
BENJAMIN (Hebrew) *Son of the right hand: fortunate*, Mar. 31
BENNETT *a form of Benedict*, Mar. 21
BERNARD (German) *Brave warrior*, Aug. 20
BERNARDO *a form of Bernard*, Aug. 20
BERNHARD *a form of Bernard*, Aug. 20
BERTON *a form of Bertrand*, Sept. 6
BERTRAN *a form of Bertrand*, Sept. 6
BERTRAND (German) *Bright raven*, Sept. 6
BONAVENTURE (Latin) *Good luck*, July 14
BONIFACE (Latin) *Doer of good*, Mar. 14
BORIS (Latin) *Roman*, July 24
BOSWELL (Latin-Teutonic) *From the cow's well*, Feb. 23
BOWEN *a form of Owen*, Mar. 3
BRANDAN (German) *From the flaming hill*, Jan. 11
BRENDAN (Celtic) *Sword*, May 16
BRODERICK *a form of Roderick*, Mar. 13
BRUCE *a form of Ambrose*, July 19
BRUNO (German) *Of dark complexion*, May 27

CARL *a form of Charles*, Mar. 2
CARLOS *a form of Charles*, Mar. 2
CARLTON *a form of Charles*, Mar. 2
CASPAR *a form of Gaspar*, Dec. 29
CECIL (Latin) *Of poor sight*, June 3

CHAD (Celtic) *The marshal*, Mar. 2
CHARLES (German) *Man*, Mar. 2
CHARLTON *a form of Charles*, Mar. 2
CHESTER (Anglo-Saxon) *A dweller in a fort*, July 17
CHRISTIAN (Latin) *Believer in Christ*, June 12
CHRISTOPHER (Greek) *Christ-bearer*, July 25
CLARENCE (Latin) *Illustrious*, Apr. 26
CLAUDE (Latin) *Lame*, Feb. 15
CLEMENCE *a variation of Clement*, Mar. 15
CLEMENT (Latin) *Mild or merciful*, Mar. 15
COLEMAN *a form of Colman*, Feb. 18
COLMAN (Celtic) *Dove*, Feb. 18
CONRAD (German) *Able in counsel*, Apr. 14
CORNELIUS (Latin) *War-horn*, Sept. 16
CYRIL (Greek) *Lordly*, Mar. 18
CYRUS (Persian) *Sun*, Jan. 31

DAMIAN (Greek) *The tamed*, Feb. 12
DAVID (Hebrew) *Beloved one*, Mar. 1
DANIEL (Hebrew) *God is my judge*, July 21
DAVIS *a form of David*, Mar. 1
DELBERT *a form of Albert*, Nov. 15
DENIS (Greek) *God of Nysa*, Oct. 9
DIXON *a form of Benedict*, Mar. 21
DOMINIC (Latin) *The Lord's*, Aug. 4
DOMINICK *a form of Dominic*, Aug. 4
DONALD (Celtic) *Dark stranger*, July 15

EARL (Anglo-Saxon) *Nobleman*, Aug. 26
EBERHARD (German) *Boar*, June 22
EDGAR (Anglo-Saxon) *Protector*, July 8
EDMOND *a form of Edmund*, Dec. 1
EDMUND (Anglo-Saxon) *Prosperous protector*, Dec. 1
EDSON *a form of Edward*, Oct. 13
EDWARD (Anglo-Saxon) *Valuable friend*, Oct. 12
EDWIN *a form of Edward*, Oct. 12

EGBERT (German) *Formidably brilliant*, Apr. 24

ELI *a form of Elias*, July 20

ELIAS (Hebrew) *Jehovah is God*, July 20

ELIJAH *a form of Elias*, July 20

ELIOT *a form of Elias*, July 20

ELLIS *a form of Elias*, July 20

ELLISON *a form of Elias*, July 20

ELMER (Anglo-Saxon) *Noble*, Aug. 25

ELSON *a form of Elias*, July 20

EMELIN *a form of Emilian*, Nov. 12

EMERSON *a form of Emilian*, Nov. 12

EMERY *a form of Emilian*, Nov. 12

EMIL *a form of Emilian*, Nov. 12

EMILIAN (German) *Industrious*, Nov. 12

EMMANUEL (Hebrew) *God is with us*, Sept. 17

EMMETT *a form of Emilian*, Nov. 12

EMORY *a form of Emilian*, Nov. 12

EPHREM (Hebrew) *Very fruitful*, June 18

ERIC (German) *Ever powerful or kingly*, May 18

ERICK *a form of Eric*, May 18

ERNEST (German) *Intent in purpose*, Nov. 7

ERROL *a form of Earl*, Aug. 26

EUGENE (Greek) *Well-born*, Aug. 23

EVAN *a form of Eugene*, Aug. 23

EVERETT *a form of Everhard*, June 22

EVERHARD (German) *Boar*, June 22

EZRA (Hebrew) A *form of Esdras, Help*, July 13

FABIAN (Latin) *Bean farmer*, Jan. 20

FELIX (Latin) *Fortunate*, July 14

FERDINAND (German) *Adventurous in life*, May 30

FIDEL *a form of Fidelis* (Latin) *The faithful*, Mar. 23

FRANCIS (German) *Free*, Oct. 4

FRANK *a form of Francis*, Oct. 4

FRANKLIN *a form of Francis*, Oct. 4

FRANZ *a form of Francis*, Oct. 4

FRED *a form of Frederick,* Jan. 6
FREDERIC *a form of Frederick,* Jan. 6
FREDERICK (German) *Peaceful ruler,* Jan. 6
FRITZ *a form of Frederick,* Jan. 6

GABRIEL (Hebrew) *God is my strength,* Sept. 14
GARCIA *a form of Gerald,* Oct. 12
GARY *a form of Gerald,* Oct. 12
GASPAR (Persian) *Treasure master,* Dec. 29
GEOFFREY *a form of Godfrey,* Jan. 13
GEORGE (Greek) *Farmer or husbandman,* Apr. 23
GERALD (German) *Mighty with the spear,* Oct. 12
GERARD (German) *Brave with the spear,* June 6
GILBERT (German) *Illustrious pledge, or hostage,* Feb. 4
GILBURT *a form of Gilbert,* Feb. 4
GILES (Greek) *Bearer of the shield,* Apr. 23
GILFORD *a form of Julius,* Apr. 12
GILL *a form of Julius,* Apr. 12
GODFREY (German) *God's peace,* Jan. 13
GORDON (Old English) *From the cornered hill,* Jan. 3
GREGORY (Greek) *Watchman,* Mar. 12
GUY (Celtic) *Guide,* June 16

HAMLIN *a form of Henry,* Mar. 2
HANS *a form of John,* Dec. 27
HAROLD (German) *Mighty in battle,* Mar. 25
HARRISON *a form of Harold,* Mar. 25
HARRY *a form of Harold,* Mar. 25
HARVEY (Celtic) *The progressive,* June 1
HENRY (German) *Ruler of the home,* Mar. 2
HERBERT (German) *Bright warrior,* Aug. 20
HERMAN (German) *A warrior,* Dec. 23
HILARY (Latin) *Cheerful,* Jan. 14
HOWARD (German) *Chief guardian,* Dec. 29
HUBERT (German) *Bright-minded,* Nov. 3
HUGH (German) *Intelligent,* Apr. 29
HUMPHREY (German) *Supporter of peace,* Mar. 8

IGNACE *a form of Ignatius,* July 31
IGNATIUS (Latin) *Ardent or fiery,* July 31
IRVIN *a form of Urban,* May 25
IRVING *a form of Urban,* May 25
ISAAC (Hebrew) *He who laughs,* Mar. 16
ISODORE (Greek) *Gift of Isis,* Jan. 15
IVAN (Hebrew) *God's gracious gift,* June 24

JACOB *a form of James,* Aug. 28
JAMES (Hebrew) *The supplanter,* July 25
JASON (Greek) *The healer,* July 12
JEFFREY *a form of Godfrey,* Jan. 13
JEREMIAS (Hebrew) *Annointed, or exalted of the Lord,* May 1
JEREMY *a form of Jeremias,* May 1
JEROME (Greek) *Of sacred name,* Sept. 30
JOACHIM (Hebrew) *The Lord will judge,* Aug. 16
JOEL (Hebrew) *Jehovah is God,* July 13
JOHN (Hebrew) *God's gracious gift,* Dec. 27
JOHNSON *a variation of John,* Dec. 27
JON *a form of John,* Dec. 27
JONAS (Hebrew) *Dove,* Sept. 21
JOSE *a form of Joseph,* Mar. 19
JOSEPH (Hebrew) *He shall add,* Mar. 19
JULES *a form of Julian,* Feb. 12
JULIAN (Greek) *Youthful,* Feb. 12
JUSTIN (Latin) *The just, or upright,* Apr. 14

KARL *a form of Charles,* Mar. 2
KENNETH (Celtic) *Comely,* Aug. 1
KENNY *a form of Kenneth,* Aug. 1
KENT (Celtic) *Head chief,* Jan. 14
KERMIT (Celtic) *Son of Dermott,* Jan. 18
KEVIN (Celtic) *Kind or gentle,* June 3
KONRAD *a form of Conrad,* Apr. 14

LANCELOT (Latin) *Man-servant,* June 27
LANCE *a form of Lancelot,* June 27

LARS *a form of Laurence,* Feb. 2
LAURENCE (Latin) *The laurel,* Feb. 2
LAWRENCE *a form of Laurence,* Feb. 2
LAZARUS (Hebrew) *Grace,* June 21
LEO (Latin) *The lion,* Apr. 11
LEON *a form of Leo,* Apr. 11
LEONARD (German) *Strong or brave as a lion,* Nov. 18
LEOPOLD (German) *Bold for the people—patriotic,* Apr. 2
LESTER *a form of Silvester,* Dec. 31
LEWIS *a form of Louis,* Apr. 28
LIONEL *a form of Leonard,* Nov. 18
LOREN *a form of Laurence,* Feb. 2
LORENZ *a form of Laurence,* Feb. 2
LORENZO *a form of Laurence,* Feb. 2
LORIN *a form of Laurence,* Feb. 2
LOUIS (German) *Famous in battle,* Apr. 28
LUCAS *a form of Luke,* Oct. 4
LUCIAN (Latin) *Light,* Jan. 7
LUCIEN *a form of Lucian,* Jan. 7
LUCIUS *a form of Luke,* Mar. 4
LUKE (Latin) *Light,* Oct. 4

MAGNUS (Latin) *Great,* Sept. 6
MANUEL (Hebrew) *God with us,* June 17
MARC *a form of Mark,* Apr. 25
MARIO *a form of Marius,* Jan. 19
MARIUS (Latin) *Martial,* Jan. 19
MARK (Latin) *Hammer,* Apr. 25
MARTIN (Latin) *The warlike,* Nov. 5
MARVIN *a form of Martin,* Nov. 5
MATHIAS *a form of Matthew,* Sept. 21
MATTHEW (Hebrew) *Gift of God,* Sept. 21
MAURICE (Latin) *Dark-skinned,* Oct. 13
MAX (Latin) *The greatest,* Oct. 12
MICHAEL (Hebrew) *Like unto the Lord,* May 14
MILES (Greek) *A mill,* Apr. 30
MITCHELL *a form of Michael,* May 14

MORGAN (Celtic) *Sea protector*, Aug. 12
MORRIS *a variation of Maurice*, Oct. 13
MOSES (Greek) *Drawn from the water*, Sept. 4
MYRON (Greek) *Fragrant*, Aug. 17

NATHAN (Hebrew) *The given*, Dec. 29
NATHANIEL *a form of Nathan*, Dec. 29
NEAL *a form of Cornelius*, Sept. 16
NELSON *a form of Cornelius*, Sept. 16
NICHOLAS (Greek) *The people's victory*, Dec. 6
NICOLAS *a form of Nicholas*, Dec. 6
NILES *a form of Nicholas*, Dec. 6
NOEL (French) *Christmas*, Sept. 26
NORBERT (German) *Njord's brightness*, June 6

OLIVER (Latin) *The olive*, July 11
OSCAR (Celt) *Bounding warrior*, Feb. 3
OSWALD (German) *Of God-like power*, Feb. 28
OTTO (German) *Prosperous or wealthy*, July 2
OWEN (Celtic) *Young warrior*, Mar. 3

PATRICK (Latin) *Noble or patrician*, Mar. 17
PAUL (Latin) *Little*, June 29
PAYTON *a form of Patrick*, Mar. 17
PEDRO *a form of Peter*, June 29
PERCY (Greek) *The destroyer*, Nov. 14
PERRY *a form of Peter*, June 29
PETER (Greek) *A rock*, June 29
PEYTON *a form of Patrick*, Mar. 17
PHILIP (Greek) *Lover of horses*, May 1
PIERCE *a form of Peter*, June 29
PIERSON *a form of Peter*, June 29

QUENTIN (Latin) *Fifth*, Oct. 4

RALPH (German) *Shield wolf*, Dec. 1
RAMON *a variation of Raymund*, July 3

RANDALL *a form of Raymund,* July 3
RAYMOND *a form of Raymund,* July 3
RAYMUND (German) *Mighty or wise protector,* July 3
RAYNALD (German) *Of firm judgment,* Feb. 9
REGINALD (German) *Of mighty or wise power,* Feb. 1
RENATO (Latin) *Reborn,* Nov. 12
REX *a form of Reginald,* Feb. 1
RICHARD (German) *Powerful ruler,* Aug. 22
ROBERT (German) *Of shining fame,* May 13
ROBIN *a form of Robert,* May 13
RODERICK (German) *Rich in fame,* Mar. 13
ROGER (German) *Famous spearman,* Mar. 1
ROLAND (German) *Fame of the land,* June 16
ROLLIN *a form of Rudolph,* Oct. 17
RONALD (German) *Of mighty power,* Aug. 20
RORY *a form of Roger,* Mar. 1
ROY *a form of Rufus,* Nov. 7
RUDOLF *a form of Rudolph,* Oct. 17
RUDOLPH (German) *Far-famed wolf,* Oct. 17
RUFUS (Latin) *Red-haired,* Nov. 7
RUPERT (German) *Bright fame,* Mar. 17

SAMSON (Hebrew) *Like the sun, resplendent,* July 28
SAMPSON *a form of Samson,* July 28
SAMUEL (Hebrew) *Asked of God,* Aug. 20
SARGENT *a form of Sergius,* Feb. 24
SEAN *a form of John,* Dec. 27
SEBASTIAN (Greek) *The revered,* Feb. 25
SERGE *a form of Sergius,* Feb. 24
SERGIUS (Latin) *To serve,* Feb. 24
SEYMOUR *a form of Maurice,* Jan. 15
SHAWN *a form of John,* Dec. 27
SIGFRID (German) *Conquering peace,* Feb. 15
SILAS *a form of Silvester,* Dec. 31
SILVESTER (Latin) *Forest dweller,* Dec. 31
SIMEON *a form of Simon,* Dec. 4
SIMON (Hebrew) *Heard,* Dec. 4

SOLOMON (Hebrew) *Peaceful,* June 25
STANLEY (Slavonic) *Glory of the camp,* Aug. 15
STEFAN *a form of Stephen,* Dec. 26
STEPHEN (Greek) *A crown or garland,* Dec. 26
STEVEN *a form of Stephen,* Dec. 26
SIDNEY (Phoenician) *The enchanter,* Dec. 10
SYDNEY *a form of Sidney,* Dec. 10
SYLVESTER *a form of Silvester,* Dec. 31

TERENCE (Latin) *Tender,* June 21
TERRIS *a form of Terence,* June 21
THADDEUS (Hebrew) *Praising God,* Nov. 24
THEODORE (Greek) *Divine gift,* Sept. 19
THOMAS (Hebrew) *The twin,* Mar. 7
TIMOTHY (Greek) *Honoring God,* Jan. 24
TOBIAS (Hebrew) *The Lord is my good,* Nov. 2

URBAN (Latin) *From the town,* May 25

VANCE *a form of Vincent,* Apr. 5
VICTOR (Latin) *The conquering,* Sept. 16
VINCENT (Latin) *Conquering,* Apr. 5
VIVIAN (Latin) *To live,* Aug. 28
VLADIMIR (Slavonic) *World ruler,* July 15

WALTER (German) *Mighty warrior,* June 4
WARD *a form of Edward,* Oct. 13
WARREN (German) *Protecting friend,* Feb. 6
WATSON *a form of Walter,* June 4
WENDEL (German) *A wanderer,* Oct. 21
WERNER (German) *A defender,* Apr. 19
WILBUR *a form of Gilbert,* Feb. 4
WILFRED *a form of Wilfrid,* Oct. 12
WILFRID (German) *Resolute for peace,* Oct. 12
WILLIAM (German) *Resolute protector,* May 28
WILLIS *a form of William,* May 28
WILSON *a form of William,* May 28

WYATT *a form of Guy,* June 16
WYLIE *a form of William,* May 28

ZACHARY (Hebrew) *Remembered by the Lord,* Nov. 5

GIRLS' NAMES

ABELLA *feminine of Abel,* Jan. 2
ADA (German) *Happy or prosperous,* Dec. 4
ADAMINA *feminine of Adam,* Dec. 24
ADELAIDE (German) *Of noble birth, cheerful,* June 15
ADELA (German) *Noble cheer,* Feb. 24
ADELE *a form of Adelaide,* June 15
ADELINA (German) *Noble,* Oct. 20
ADELINE *a form of Adelaide,* June 15
ADRIENNE *feminine of Adrian,* Jan. 9
AGATHA (Greek) *Good,* Feb. 5
AGATHE *a form of Agatha,* Feb. 5
AGNES (Greek) *Sacred and pure,* Jan. 21
AILEEN *a form of Helen,* Aug. 18
AIMEE (French) *Beloved,* June 10
ALBERTA (German) *Noble brightness,* Mar. 11
ALBERTINA *a form of Alberta,* Mar. 11
ALDA (German) *Rich,* Apr. 26
ALEXANDRA *feminine of Alexander,* Mar. 18
ALEXIA (Greek) *Helper of mankind,* June 29
ALEXIS *a form of Alexia,* June 29
ALICE *a form of Adelaide,* June 15
ALICIA *a form of Adelaide,* June 15
ALISA *a form of Adelaide,* June 15
ALISON *a form of Louise,* Mar. 15
ALMA (Latin) *Fair and sweet,* Aug. 15
ALPHONSA *feminine of Alphonsus,* Aug. 7
AMALIA (Rom.) *Industrious, a form of Amalburga,* July 10

AMANDA *feminine of Amandus*, Oct. 15

AMELIA *a form of Amalia*, July 10

AMY *a form of Amata, Loved*, July 10

ANASTASIA (Greek) *One who shall rise again*, Mar. 10

ANDREA *feminine of Andrew*, Nov. 20

ANGELA (Greek) *Angelic*, May 31

ANGELICA *a form of Angela*, May 31

ANGELINA (Greek) *Like an angel*, July 15

ANGELINE *a form of Angelina*, July 15

ANITA *a form of Anne*, July 26

ANN a form of Anna, Sept. 1

ANNA (Hebrew) *Prayer*, Sept. 1

ANNABELLE *a form of Anne*, July 26

ANNE (Hebrew) *Mercy, grace*, July 26

ANNETTE *a form of Anne*, July 26

ANTOINETTE (Latin) *Beyond praise*, Feb. 28

ARNOLDINE *feminine of Arnold*, July 8

ATHANASIA (Greek) *Immortal*, Aug. 14

AUDREY *a form of Ethel*, June 23

AUGUSTA (Latin) *The most exalted*, Mar. 27

AVA (Latin) *Bird*, Apr. 29

BABETTE *a form of Barbara*, Dec. 4

BARBARA (Greek) *Stranger*, Dec. 4

BASILIA *feminine of Basil*, June 14

BEATRICE *a form of Beatrix*, Aug. 18

BEATRIX (Latin) *She who blesses others*, Aug. 18

BELINA (Italian) *Serpent-like*, Feb. 19

BENEDICTA (Latin) *The blessed*, May 6

BENITA *a form of Benedicta*, May 6

BERENICE (Greek) *Bringer of victory*, Oct. 4

BERDINE *a form of Bertha*, July 4

BERNADENE *a form of Bernadette*, Apr. 16

BERNADETTE (German) *Firm bear*, Apr. 16

BERNADINE *a form of Bernadette*, Apr. 16

BERNETTE *a form of Bernadette*, Apr. 16

BERNICE *a form of Berenice*, Oct. 4

BERNITA *a form of Bernadette*, Apr. 16

BERTA *a form of Bertha*, July 4

BERTHA (German) *Bright, glorious*, July 4

BERTHE *a form of Bertha*, July 4

BERTINA *a form of Bertha*, July 4

BESS *a form of Elizabeth*, July 8

BETH *a form of Elizabeth*, July 8

BETSY *a form of Elizabeth*, July 8

BETTE *a form of Elizabeth*, July 8

BETTINA *a form of Elizabeth*, July 8

BETTY *a form of Elizabeth*, July 8

BEVERLY *a feminine name derived from the surname of St. John of Beverley*, May 7

BIANCA *a form of Blanche*, July 5

BLANCH *a form of Blanche*, July 5

BLANCHE (German) *White or fair*, July 5

BONNIE *feminine of Boniface*, Mar. 14

BRENDA *feminine of Brendan*, May 16

BRIDGET *a form of Brigid*, Oct. 8

BRIGID (Celtic) *Great strength*, Oct. 8

BRIDGIT *a form of Brigid*, Oct. 8

BRIGITTE *a form of Brigid*, Oct. 8

CAMILLA (Etruscan) *Attendant at a sacrifice*, May 31

CAMILLE *a form of Camilla*, May 31

CANDIDA (Latin) *White*, Sept. 4

CANDIDE *a form of Candida*, Sept. 4

CARLOTTA *feminine of Charles*, Mar. 2

CARMEN (Latin) *Rosy*, Aug. 15

CAROL *a form of Catherine*, Dec. 31

CAROLINA *feminine of Charles*, Mar. 2

CAROLINE *feminine of Charles*, Mar. 2

CAROLYN *feminine of Charles*, Mar. 2

CARRIE *a form of Catherine*, Dec. 31

CATHERINE (Greek) *Pure, spotless*, Dec. 31

CECILA (Latin) *Blind*, Nov. 22

CECILIA *a form of Cecila*, Nov. 22

CELESTA (Greek) *Heavenly*, Apr. 16
CELESTE *a form of Celesta*, Apr. 16
CELIA *a form of Cecila*, Nov. 22
CELINE (Latin) *Pertaining to the heavens*, Oct. 21
CHARITY *a Christian virtue*, Aug. 1
CHARLENE *feminine of Charles*, Mar. 2
CHARLOTTE *feminine of Charles*, Mar. 2
CHERYL *feminine of Charles*, Mar. 2
CHRISTA *a form of Christiana*, Jan. 18
CHRISTIANA (Greek) *The Christian or anointed*, Jan. 18
CHRISTINE *a form of Christiana*, Jan. 18
CLAIRE *a form of Clare*, Aug. 12
CLARA *a form of Clare*, Aug. 12
CLARE (Latin) *Shiny or distinguished*, Aug. 12
CLARISSA *a form of Clare*, Aug. 12
CLAUDETTE *a form of Claudia*, Aug. 7
CLAUDIA (Latin) *Lame*, Aug. 7
CLAUDINA *a form of Claudia*, Aug. 7
CLAUDINE *a form of Claudia*, Aug. 7
CLEMENTINE *feminine of Clement*, Mar. 15
CLOTILDE (German) *Distinguished warrioress*, June 3
COLLETTA *a form of Colette*, Mar. 6
COLETTE (French-Latin) *Necklace*, Mar. 6
CONSTANCE (Latin) *Firm*, Sept. 19
CORA *a form of Cordelia*, Oct. 22
CORDELIA (Latin) *Warmhearted*, Oct. 22
CORNELIA (Latin) *Horn*, Mar. 31
CYNTHIA (Greek) *The moon*, Feb. 8

DANIELLE *feminine of Daniel*, July 21
DANITA *feminine of Daniel*, July 21
DEANNA *a form of Diana*, July 10
DELIA *a form of Cordelia*, Oct. 22
DELLA *a form of Adela*, Feb. 24
DIANA (Latin) *Divine moon*, June 10
DIANE *a form of Diana*, June 10
DIXIE *a form of Benedicta*, May 6

DOLLY *a form of Dorothy*, Feb. 6

DOLORES *a name used in connection with the Blessed Virgin*, Aug. 15.

DONNA *a form of Donata*, Dec. 31

DORA *a form of Dorothy*, Feb. 6

DORETTE *a form of Dorothy*, Feb. 6

DORINDA *a form of Dorothy*, Feb. 6

DORIS *a form of Dorothy*, Feb. 6

DOROTHEA *a form of Dorothy*, Feb. 6

DOROTHY (Greek) *Gift of God*, Feb. 6

EDA *a form of Edith*, Sept. 16

EDLINE *a form of Adelaide*, June 15

EDITA *a form of Edith*, Sept. 16

EDITH (German) *Rich gift*, Sept. 16

EDITHA *a form of Edith*, Sept. 16

EDMEE *feminine of Edmund*, Dec. 1

EDMONIA *feminine of Edmund*, Dec. 1

EDNA *feminine of Edwin*, Oct. 12

EDWINA *feminine of Edwin*, Oct. 12

EDYTHE *a form of Edith*, Sept. 16

EILEEN *a form of Helen*, Aug. 18

ELAINE *a form of Helen*, Aug. 18

ELEANOR *a form of Helen*, Aug. 18

ELEANORA *a form of Helen*, Aug. 18

ELINOR *a form of Helen*, Aug. 18

ELISA *a form of Elizabeth*, July 8

ELISABETH *a form of Elizabeth*, July 8

ELIZABETH (Hebrew) *Consecrated to God*, July 8

ELLA *a form of Helen*, Aug. 18

ELLEN *a form of Helen*, Aug. 18

ELOISE *a form of Louise*, Mar. 15

ELSA *a form of Adelaide*, June 15

ELSIE *a form of Adelaide*, June 15

EMELDA *a form of Imelda*, May 12

EMELINA *a form of Emily*, Sept. 19

EMELINE *a form of Emily*, Sept. 19

EMILIE *a form of Emily*, Sept. 19

EMILY (German-Latin) *Hard-working*, Sept. 19
EMMA (German) *Energetic and hard-working*, June 17
ESTELLE *a form of Esther*, Dec. 20
ESTHER (Persian) *Star*, Dec. 20
ETHEL (German) *Noble*, June 23
EUGENIA (Greek) *The well-born*, Dec. 25
EUGENIE *a form of Eugenia*, Dec. 25
EUNICE *Happy victory*, Oct. 28
EVA (Hebrew) *Life*, May 26
EVE *a form of Eva*, May 26
EVELINE *a form of Eva*, May 26
EVELYN *a form of Eva*, May 26

FAITH (Latin) *The believing or faithful*, Oct. 6
FAY *a form of Faith*, Oct. 6
FAYE *a form of Faith*, Oct. 6
FELICE *a form of Felicia*, Oct. 5
FELICIA (Latin) *One who is fortunate*, Oct. 5
FELICITAS (Latin) *Happiness*, Mar. 26
FELISE *a form of Felicia*, Oct. 5
FERNANDA *feminine of Ferdinand*, May 30
FLEUR *a form of Flora*, July 11
FLORA (Latin) *A flower*, June 11
FLORENCE (Latin) *Blooming, flourishing*, Nov. 10
FLORIS *a form of Flora*, June 11
FRANCES (German) *Free*, Mar. 9
FRANCESCA *a form of Frances*, Mar. 9
FRANCINE *a form of Frances*, Mar. 9
FRANCISCA *a form of Frances*, Mar. 9
FREDA *feminine of Frederick*, Jan. 9
FRIEDA *feminine of Frederick*, Jan. 9

GABRIELLA *a form of Gabrielle*, Oct. 17
GABRIELLE (Hebrew) *God is my strength*, Oct. 17
GENEVIEVE (Celtic) *White wave*, Jan. 3
GEORGETTE *a form of Georgia*, Feb. 15
GEORGIA (Greek) *Earth worker*, Feb. 15

GEORGIANA *a form of Georgia,* Feb. 15
GEORGINA *a form of Georgia,* Feb. 15
GERALDINE *feminine of Gerald,* Oct. 12
GERMAINE *a form of Germana,* June 15
GERMANA (Latin) *A German,* June 15
GERTRUDE (German) *Spear maiden,* Nov. 16
GINA *a form of Regina,* Sept. 2
GINGER *a form of Virginia,* Aug. 15
GISELLE *a form of Elizabeth,* July 8
GLADYS (Latin) *Lame,* Mar. 29
GRACE *a form of Anne,* July 26
GRETA *a form of Margaret,* Feb. 3
GRETCHEN *a form of Margaret,* Feb. 3
GWEN (Celtic) *The white or fair,* Oct. 18
GWENDOLEN (Celtic) *White-browed,* Mar. 28
GWENDOLINE *a form of Gwendolen,* Mar. 28
GWYN *a form of Gwen,* Oct. 18
GWYNNE *a form of Gwen,* Oct. 18

HADASSAH *a form of Esther,* Dec. 20
HANNAH *a form of Anne,* July 26
HARRIET *feminine of Harold,* Mar. 25
HAZEL *a form of Eva,* May 26
HEDDA *a form of Hedwig,* Feb. 28
HEDWIG (German) *Refuge in battle,* Feb. 28
HEDY *a form of Hedwig,* Feb. 28
HELEN (Greek) *Light,* Aug. 18
HELENA *a form of Helen,* Aug. 18
HELENE *a form of Helen,* Aug. 18
HELGA *a form of Olga,* July 18
HENRIETTA *feminine of Harold,* Mar. 25
HERMIONE (Greek) *Of the Earth,* Sept. 4
HESTER *a form of Esther,* Dec. 20
HILDA (German) *A warrioress,* Nov. 17
HILDEGARD (German) *A protecting warrioress,* Sept. 17
HILDEGARDE *a form of Hildegard,* Sept. 17
HONORA *a form of Honoria,* Sunday after Easter

HONORIA (Latin) *Honorable,* Sunday after Easter
HOPE *a theological virtue,* Aug. 1
HYACINTHA (Latin) *The hyacinth,* Jan. 20

IDA (German) *Happy,* Apr. 13
ILKA *a form of Emily,* Sept. 19
ILSA *a form of Adela,* Feb. 24
IMELDA (Latin) *An image,* May 12
IMOGENE *a form of Imelda,* May 12
INA *a form of Ines,* Jan. 21
INES (Greek) *Pure, gentle, meek,* Jan. 21
INEZ *a form of Agnes,* Jan. 21
IRENE (Greek) *Peace,* Oct. 20
ISABEL *a form of Isabelle,* Feb. 26
ISABELLA *a form of Isabelle,* Feb. 26
ISABELLE (Hebrew) *Consecrated to God,* Feb. 26
ISOBEL *a form of Isabelle,* Feb. 26

JACINTA *a form of Hyacintha,* Jan. 20
JACQUELINE *feminine of James,* July 25
JANE (Hebrew) *Gift of God,* Aug. 21
JANET *a form of Jane,* Aug. 21
JANETTE *a form of Jane,* Aug. 21
JANICE *a form of Jane,* Aug. 21
JAYNE *a form of Jane,* Aug. 21
JEAN *a form of Joanna* May 24
JEANETTE *a form of Joanna,* May 24
JEANNE *a form of Joanna,* May 24
JENNIFER *a form of Joanna,* May 24
JENNY *a form of Joanna,* May 24
JESSICA *a form of Joanna,* May 24
JESSIE *a form of Joanna,* May 24
JILL *a form of Julia,* May 22
JILLIAN *a form of Julia,* May 22
JOAN (Hebrew) *God's gracious gift,* May 30
JOANNA (Hebrew) *God's gracious gift,* May 24
JOCELYN *feminine of Justin,* Apr. 14

JOHANNA *a form of Jane*, Aug. 21
JOSEPHINE *feminine of Joseph*, Mar. 19
JOY *a form of Jucunda*, Nov. 25
JOYCE *a form of Jucunda*, Nov. 25
JUANITA *a form of Joanna*, May 24
JUCUNDA (Latin) *Joyful*, Nov. 25
JUDITH (Hebrew) *Praised*, Sept. 14
JUDITHE *a form of Judith*, Sept. 14
JUDY *a form of Judith*, Sept. 14
JULIA (Greek) *Youthful*, May 22
JULIANA (Greek) *Youthful*, Feb. 7
JULIENNE *a form of Julia*, May 22
JULIET *a form of Julia*, May 22
JULIETTE (Greek) *Youthful*, July 17
JUSTINA *feminine of Justin*, Apr. 14
JUSTINE *feminine of Justin*, Apr. 14

KAREN *a form of Catherine*, Dec. 31
KATE *a form of Catherine*, Dec. 31
KATHLEEN *a form of Catherine*, Dec. 31
KATHRYN *a form of Catherine*, Dec. 31
KATRINA *a form of Catherine*, Dec. 31
KATRINE *a form of Catherine*, Dec. 31
KAY *a form of Catherine*, Dec. 31
KITTY *a form of Catherine*, Dec. 31

LANA *feminine of Alan*, Oct. 26
LAURA (Latin) *The Laurel*, Oct. 19
LAUREEN *a form of Laura*, Oct. 19
LAUREL *a form of Laura*, Oct. 19
LAURETTA *a form of Laura*, Oct. 19
LAURETTE *a form of Laura*, Oct. 19
LEA (Hebrew) *Weary*, Mar. 22
LEE *a form of Elizabeth*, July 8
LEIGH *a form of Lea*, Mar. 22
LEILA *a form of Lelia*, Aug. 11
LELA *a form of Lelia*, Aug. 11

LELAH *a form of Lelia,* Aug. 11
LELIA (Arabic) *Darkness,* Aug. 11
LENA *a form of Helen,* Aug. 18
LENORA *a form of Helen,* Aug. 18
LENORE *a form of Helen,* Aug. 18
LEONA *feminine of Leo,* Apr. 11
LEONORE *a form of Helen,* Aug. 18
LILLIAN *a form of Elizabeth,* July 8
LILLY *a form of Elizabeth,* July 8
LINA *feminine of Charles,* Mar. 2
LISA *a form of Elizabeth,* July 8
LISETTE *a form of Louise,* Mar. 15
LIZA *a form of Elizabeth,* July 8
LOIS *a form of Louise,* Mar. 15
LOLA *feminine of Charles,* Mar. 2
LOLANDA *feminine of Charles,* Mar. 2
LOLITA *feminine of Charles,* Mar. 2
LORALIE *a form of Laura,* Oct. 19
LORETTA *a form of Laura,* Oct. 19
LORNA *a form of Laura,* Oct. 19
LORRAINE *a form of Laura,* Oct. 19
LOTTY *feminine of Charles,* Mar. 2
LOUELLA *a form of Louise,* Mar. 15
LOUISA *a form of Louise,* Mar. 15
LOUISE (German) *Renowned in war,* Mar. 15
LUCIA *a form of Lucy,* Dec. 13
LUCIANA *a form of Lucy,* Dec. 13
LUCILLE *a form of Lucy,* Dec. 13
LUCINDA *a form of Lucy,* Dec. 13
LUCRETIA (Latin) *Bringer of light,* Nov. 23
LUCY (Latin) *Light,* Dec. 13
LULU *a form of Louise,* Mar. 15
LYDIA (Greek) *From Lydia,* Aug. 3
LYNN (Anglo-Saxon) *A Cascade—a form of Ermalinda,* Feb. 13

MABEL (Latin) *Amiable,* July 13
MADELEINE (Hebrew) *The Tower,* May 25

MADELINE *a form of Madeleine,* May 25
MADGE *a form of Margaret,* Feb. 3
MAE *a form of Mary,* Aug. 15
MAGDA *a form of Madeleine,* May 25
MAGDALEN *a form of Madeleine,* May 25
MAISIE *a form of Margaret,* Feb. 3
MAMIE *a form of Mary,* Aug. 15
MANUELA *feminine of Manuel,* June 17
MARCELLA (Latin) *Belonging to Mars,* Jan. 31
MARCELLINA *a form of Marcella,* Jan. 31
MARCELLINE *a form of Marcella,* Jan. 31
MARCIA *feminine of Mark,* Apr. 25
MARET *a form of Mary,* Aug. 15
MARGARET (Greek) *A pearl,* Feb. 3
MARGARETA *a form of Margaret,* Feb. 3
MARGARETTA *a form of Margaret,* Feb. 3
MARGARITA *a form of Margaret,* Feb. 3
MARGERY *a form of Margaret,* Feb. 3
MARGOT *a form of Margaret,* Feb. 3
MARGUERITE *a form of Margaret,* Feb. 3
MARIA *a form of Mary,* Aug. 15
MARIAN *a form of Mary,* Aug. 15
MARIANA (Hebrew) *Bitter grace,* Apr. 27
MARIANNA *a form of Mariana,* Apr. 27
MARIANNE *a form of Mariana,* Apr. 27
MARIE *a form of Mary,* Aug. 15
MARIETTA *a form of Mary,* Aug. 15
MARILYN *a form of Mary,* Aug. 15
MARINA (Latin) *Maiden of the sea,* June 18
MARJORIE *a form of Margaret,* Feb. 3
MARLENE *a form of Madeleine,* May 25
MARTHA (Hebrew) *Lady or Mistress,* June 29
MARTINA (Latin) *Warlike,* Jan. 30
MARTINE *a form of Martina,* Jan. 30
MARY (Hebrew) *Bitterness,* Aug. 15
MARYANN *a form of Mariana,* Apr. 27
MATHILDA *a form of Matilda,* Mar. 14

MATHILDE *a form of Matilda,* Mar. 14
MATILDA (German) *Mighty in battle,* Mar. 14
MAUD *a form of Mary,* Aug. 15
MAURA (Latin) *Dark,* Nov. 30
MAUREEN *a form of Mary,* Aug. 15
MAXINE *feminine of Max,* Oct. 12
MELANIA (Greek) *Darkness,* June 8
MELANIE *a form of Melania,* June 8
MERCEDES *a form of Mary,* Aug. 15
MICHELE *feminine of Michael,* May 14
MILDRED (Anglo-Saxon) *Mild or gentle counselor,* July 13
MILDRID *a form of Mildred,* July 13
MIMI *feminine of William,* May 28
MINNIE *a form of Mary,* Aug. 15
MIRIAM *a form of Mary,* Aug. 15
MOIRA *a form of Mary,* Aug. 15
MOLLY *a form of Mary,* Aug. 15
MONA *a form of Monica,* May 4
MONICA (Latin) *Advisor,* May 4
MONIQUE *a form of Monica,* May 4
MURIEL *a form of Mary,* Aug. 15
MYRTLE *a form of Mary,* Aug. 15

NADA *a form of Hope,* Aug. 1
NADINE *a form of Hope,* Aug. 1
NAN *a form of Anna,* Sept. 1
NANA *a form of Anne,* July 26
NANCY *a form of Anna,* Sept. 1
NANETTE *a form of Anna,* Sept. 1
NATALIA (Latin) *Christmas child,* Dec. 1
NATALIE *a form of Natalia,* Dec. 1
NATHALIE *a form of Natalia,* Dec. 1
NEDA *feminine of Edward,* Oct. 13
NELLIE *a form of Helen,* Aug. 18
NETTIE *a form of Antonia* (Latin: The inestimable) Feb. 28
NICOLETTE *feminine of Nicholas,* Dec. 6
NINA *a form of Anne,* July 26

NORA *a form of Helen*, Aug. 18
NOREEN *a form of Honoria*, Low Sunday.

OCTAVIA (Latin) *Eighth born*, Apr. 15
ODETTA *a form of Odile*, Dec. 13
ODILE (German) *Happy battle maid*, Dec. 13
OLGA (German) *Holy*, July 11
OLIVA (Latin) *The olive*, June 3
OLIVE *a form of Oliva*, June 3
OLIVIA *a form of Oliva*, June 3
OSWALDA *feminine of Oswald*, Feb. 28

PAMELA *a form of Helen*, Aug. 18
PATRICIA (Latin) *Well-born*, Aug. 25
PAULA (Latin) *Little*, June 11
PAULETTE *a form of Paula*, June 11
PAULINA (Latin) *Little*, Mar. 14
PAULINE *a form of Paula*, June 11
PAULITA *a form of Paula*, June 11
PEARL *a form of Margaret*, Feb. 3
PHEBE *a form of Phoebe*, Sept. 3
PHILIPPA (Greek) *Lover of horses*, Sept. 20
PHOEBE (Greek) *Shining, brilliant*, Sept. 3
PILAR *a form of Mary*, Aug. 15
POLLY *a form of Mary*, Aug. 15
PRISCILLA (Latin) *The ancient*, Jan. 16
PRUDENCE (Latin) *Wise*, May 6

RAMONA *feminine of Raymund*, July 3
REGINA (Latin) *Queen or queenly*, Sept. 7
RENATA *feminine of Renato*, Nov. 12
RENEE *feminine of Renato*, Nov. 12
RETA *a form of Rita*, May 22
RHODA *a form of Rose*, Nov. 18
RIA *a form of Mary*, Aug. 15
RITA (Greek) *The pearl*, May 22
ROBERTA *feminine of Robert*, May 13

ROSA *a form of Rose*, Nov. 18
ROSALIA *a form of Rose*, Nov. 18
ROSALIE *a form of Rose*, Nov. 18
ROSALIND *a form of Roseline*, Jan. 17
ROSALYN *a form of Roseline*, Jan. 17
ROSE (Latin) *A rose*, Nov. 18
ROSELINE (Latin) *Fair rose*, Jan. 17
ROSINA *a form of Rose*, Nov. 18

STELLA *a form of Esther*, Dec. 20
STEPHANIE *feminine of Stephen*, Dec. 26
SUSAN *a form of Susanna*, Sept. 19
SUSANNA (Hebrew) *A lily*, Sept. 19
SUSANNAH *a form of Susanna*, Sept. 19
SUSANNE *a form of Susanna*, Sept. 19
SUZANNE *a form of Susanna*, Sept. 19
SUZETTE *a form of Susanna*, Sept. 19
SYLVIA (Latin) *Bred in the country*, Nov. 3

TERESA (Greek) *The harvester*, Oct. 3
THEDA *a form of Theodora*, Apr. 1
THEODORA (Greek) *Gift of God*, Apr. 1
THELMA (Greek) *Nursling*, June 26
THERESE *a form of Teresa*, Oct. 3
THOMASINA *feminine of Thomas*, Mar. 7
TINA *a form of Christine*, Jan. 8
TONIA *a form of Antonia*, Feb. 28
TRACY *a form of Teresa*, Oct. 3
TRUDY *a form of Gertrude*, Nov. 16

URSULA (Latin) *Little she-bear*, Oct. 21

VALERIA (Latin) *Healthy*, Apr. 28
VALERIE *a form of Valeria*, Apr. 28
VERA (Latin) *True*, Jan. 24
VERONICA (Latin) *True image*, July 12
VICTORIA *femininie of Victor*, Sept. 16

VIOLA (Latin) *Violet*, May 3
VIOLET *a form of Viola*, May 3
VIOLETTE *a form of Viola*, May 3
VIRGINIA *a name used in connection with Mary, the Blessed Virgin*, Aug. 15
VIVIEN *feminine of Vivian*, Aug. 28

WANDA (German) *The wanderer*, Apr. 17
WENDY *a form of Wanda*, Apr. 17
WILHELMINA *femine of William*, May 28
WILLA *feminine of William*, May 28
WILLETTA *feminine of William*, May 28
WILMA *feminine of William*, May 28
WINIFRED (German) *Friend of peace*, Nov. 3

YOLANDE *a form of Viola*, May 3
YVETTE (Hebrew) *Praise*, Jan. 13
YVONNE *feminine of Ives—Scandinavian: Archer*, May 19

ZITA (Greek) *The harvester*, Apr. 27

8

Prayers for Expectant Mothers

A PRAYER FOR HELP TO BECOME A GOOD MOTHER

Mary, my Mother, grant that my little child may instruct me in the ways of God. Let its innocent eyes speak to me of the spotless holiness of Jesus. Let its open smile remind me of the great love God has for His creatures. Let its helplessness teach me the unbounded power of God. May its first feeble effort to speak call to my mind the wisdom of the Almighty. May its simple trust in me lead me to cherish a like confidence in God. May my love for God be stimulated by the deep-rooted affection my child has for me. May I in all these things grow in a greater appreciation of my holy motherhood. Mary, I trust in you to obtain this favor for me. Amen. Mother of Mothers, pray for me!

A PRAYER FOR THE PRIVILEGE OF MOTHERHOOD

Dearest Mother of the Infant Jesus, by that most treasured privilege of your divine Maternity, I entreat you! In the name of these holy joys you knew when in an ecstasy of love you pressed your little Baby to your breast, I implore you to hear and bless my petition! Motherhood is very dear to you, Mary. You, the Queen of Mothers and the Mother of Mothers, know as no other mother can, the exalted dignity of motherhood. You know how immensely great is the privilege to call into this world a tiny soul destined to praise God forever in heaven.

This is the blessing I ask of you, Mary! Confidently I seek it, for I know that holy motherhood is so precious in your sight. Confidently I trust in your intercession for this favor, since Jesus is the lover of little children and has said that we should allow them to come unto Him. It is this I ask of you; it is this trust I commit to your holy intercession—that I might be privileged to bring to Jesus a little one such as He so dearly loves, that He may bless it, and that He may bless me too in my motherhood, and that He may increase us always in sanctification in the fullness of His divine life. Amen. Mother of Mothers, Pray for me!

BLESSING OF AN EXPECTANT MOTHER

℣. Our help is in the name of the Lord.

℟. Who made heaven and earth.

℣. Save Thy servant, Lord.

℟. For she puts her hope, O God, in Thee.

℣. Be a tower of strength for her, O Lord.

℟. Against Enemy attack.

℣. Let not the Enemy have power against her.

℟. Nor the son of evil come near to harm her.

℣. O Lord, send her aid from Thy holy place.

℟. And guard her from Sion.

℣. O Lord, hear my prayer.

℟. And let my cry come unto Thee.

℣. The Lord be with you.

℟. And with your spirit.

Let us pray.

Almighty, everlasting God, Thou hast granted Thy servants in the profession of the true Faith, to show forth the glory of the eternal Trinity and to adore Its Unity in the power of Its Majesty. We ask that Thy servant, N., by her constancy in that Faith, may ever be safeguarded against all adversity. Through Christ our Lord.

℟. Amen.

Let us pray.

O Lord God, Creator of all, Thou art mighty and awe-inspiring, just and merciful; Thou alone art kind and loving and didst set Israel free from every evil, making our fathers Thy chosen people. Thou didst sanctify them by the power of Thy Spirit and by the co-working of the Holy Ghost didst prepare the body and soul of the glorious Virgin to become a worthy home for Thy Son. Thou didst fill John the Baptist with the Holy Ghost, making him leap with joy in his mother's womb. Accept now the offering of the contrite heart and the ardent desire of Thy servant, N., who humbly petitions Thee for the welfare of the child which Thou didst grant her to conceive. Protect the work which is Thine, and guard it from all the deceit and harm of our bitter Enemy. May the hand of Thy mercy assist her delivery, and may her child see the light of day without harm; may it be kept safe for the holy rebirth of Baptism, serve Thee always in all things, and thereby merit everlasting life. Through the same Christ our Lord.

℟. Amen.

The priest then sprinkles the woman with holy water, and prays—Psalm 66:

> May God have pity on us and bless us; *
> May He let His face shine upon us.

So may Your way be known upon the earth; *
  among all nations, Your salvation.
May the peoples praise You, O God; *
  may all the peoples praise You!
May the nations be glad and exult
  because You rule the peoples in equity; *
  the nations on the earth You guide.
May the peoples praise You, O God; *
  may all the peoples praise You.
The earth has yielded its fruits; *
  God, our God, has blessed us.
May God bless us, *
  and may all the ends of the earth fear Him!
Glory be to the Father, and to the Son, *
  and to the Holy Spirit.
As it was in the beginning, is now, and ever shall be, *
  world without end. Amen.

℣. Let us praise the Father and the Son with the Holy Spirit.
℟. Let us praise and glorify Him forever.
℣. To His angels God has given charge over you.
℟. To guard you in all your ways.
℣. O Lord, hear my prayer.
℟. And let my cry come unto Thee.
℣. The Lord be with you.
℟. And with your spirit.
Let us pray.

Visit this dwelling we beg Thee, O Lord, and drive far
from it and from this Thy servant, N., all the snares of the Enemy. May Thy holy angels dwell here to preserve her and her
child in peace, and may Thy blessing be ever upon her. Save
them, O almighty God, and bestow upon them Thy unfailing
light. Through Christ our Lord.

℟. Amen.

May the blessing of Almighty God, the Father, the Son, and

Holy Spirit, come down upon you and your child, and remain forever.

Rℐ. Amen.

A NOVENA TO OUR LADY OF A HAPPY DELIVERY

The novena may be made by saying the prayers below on nine consecutive days or weeks.

Who is she that cometh forth as the morning rising, fair as the moon, bright as the sun, terrible as an army set in battle array?

I am the Mother of Fair Love, and of fear, and of knowledge, and of holy hope.

In me is all grace of the way and of the truth; in me is all hope of life and of virtue.

Come over to me, all ye that desire me, and be filled with my fruits.

For my spirit is sweet above honey, and my inheritance above honey and the honeycomb.

My memory is unto everlasting generations.

They that eat me shall yet hunger; and they that drink me shall yet thirst.

He that hearkeneth to me shall not be confounded; and they that work by me shall not sin.

They that explain me shall have life everlasting.

Who is she that cometh forth as the morning rising, fair as the moon, bright as the sun, terrible as an army set in battle array?

I am the Mother of Fair Love, and of fear, and of knowledge, and of holy hope.

My memory is unto everlasting generations.

Let us pray.

Most tender and loving Mother Mary, in union with you I adore the divine Majesty. Whilst joyfully giving thanks to God for the wonderful graces which He conferred upon you in life, and for the great glory with which He has gifted you in Heaven, I come to you with heartfelt love, begging you to secure for me by your powerful intercession the inestimable blessing of living and dying in the state of grace. I also beseech you to obtain the favor I ask in this novena. (Mention the favor you wish to obtain.) But if what I ask is not for the glory of God or for the good of souls, do you obtain for me what is most conducive to both.

℣. Pray for us, O holy Mother Mary.

℟. That we may be made worthy of the promises of Christ.

Let us pray.

O God, who wast pleased that at the message of an angel Your Word should take flesh in the womb of the Blessed Virgin Mary, grant that we your suppliants, who believe her to be truly the Mother of God, may be helped by the prayers she on Your behalf offers to You. Through the same Jesus Christ, Your Son Our Lord, who liveth and reigneth with Thee in the unity of the Holy Ghost, God, world without end. Amen.

℣. Our Lady of Happy Delivery.

℟. Pray for us who have recourse to thee!

(—*Mother's Manual*, A. Francis Coomes, S.J., The Queen's Work, St. Louis.)

9

The Expectant Mother's Record

A section where you can list phone numbers to be called in an emergency, where you can record your progress each month and where you can write down the instructions your doctor gives you. Keeping these records will not only aid you in your present pregnancy but will serve as a valuable point of reference for any future pregnancies you may have.

Keep this book in a handy place so that you will be able to refer to it quickly, if necessary.

Family Doctor

Name _____

Address _____

Phone No. _____

Your Obstetrician

Name _____

Address _____

Phone No. _____

Night Phone _____

Pharmacy

Name _____

Address _____

Phone No. _____

Hospital

Name _____

Address _____

Phone No. _____

Taxi or Ambulance Companies

Name _____

Address _____

Phone No. _____

Name _____

Address _____

Phone No. _____

Friends and Relatives (Persons to call in an emergency)

Name _____	Name _____
Address _____	Address _____
Phone No. _____	Phone No. _____
Name _____	Name _____
Address _____	Address _____
Phone No. _____	Phone No. _____

Information the doctor should have (*List here such pertinent facts as date of last menstruation, date you first observed signs of life, etc., which the doctor will want to know about on your visit*) :

Questions to ask your doctor (*List here points you wish to discuss on your visit but which are not important enough to warrant an immediate phone call*):

Questions to ask your doctor

Questions to ask your doctor

YOUR DOCTOR'S INSTRUCTIONS

Index